Overcoming Fears and Tears

My Ostomy Story
A Journey to Wellness

Kate Murray

With Bert Crathan

First published in Australia 2024
Second edition Published by Kate Murray July 2024
Copyright © Kate Murray 2024
Email: katemurray1979@gmail.com

Cover design, typesetting: WorkingType (www.workingtype.com.au)

The right of Kate Murray to be identified as the
Author of the Work has been asserted in accordance with the
Copyright, Designs and Patents Act 1988.

All rights reserved. No part of this publication may be reproduced, stored in a retrieval system, or transmitted, in any form or by any means without the prior written permission of the publisher, nor be otherwise circulated in any form of binding or cover other than that in which it is published and without a similar condition being imposed on the subsequent purchaser.

Front and back cover photos courtesy of Spartan USA
Photographs on pages 177 & 181 courtesy of Anthony Byron Photography

ISBN: 978-0-646898-79-7

About the Author

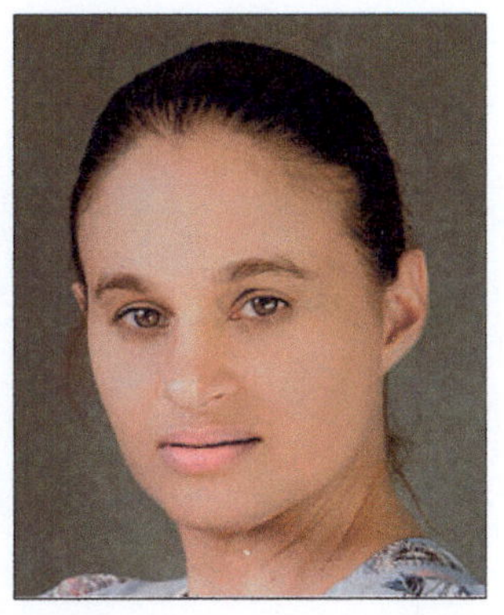

Trained initially in the hospitality sector and employed for more than twelve years in the airline industry, Kate Murray then trained as a registered nurse. This change of career was motivated by her experience of spending many long periods in hospital as a patient and appreciating the work of nurses. Kate became an advocate for those suffering from bowel diseases. Initially, she spoke at clinical workshops, with the audience comprising her peers and many senior medical staff. New avenues opened in the private sector to speak at different public forums, with direct involvement with a number of peak bodies representing people with bowel diseases.

Kate has also written articles for hospital and peak body magazines and newsletters about techniques of medical care for patients with bowel disease. Following a hiatus due to COVID-19, Kate continues her work as an advocate, underpinned by this book, *Overcoming Fears and Tears: My Ostomy Story.*

Contents

Timeline and Glossary		vi
Preface		vii
Chapter 1	The Early Years	1
Chapter 2	Early Symptoms, Surgeries and Treatments	5
Chapter 3	The Airline Experiment	13
Chapter 4	The Desperate Search for a Breakthrough	23
Chapter 5	Hard Decisions	44
Chapter 6	The Life-Changing Surgery	54
Chapter 7	A New Lease of Life and New Discoveries	64
Chapter 8	Rebooting my Career	79
Chapter 9	Training with Intent	88
Chapter 10	Preparing to Engage in a Lifelong Learning Experience	98
Chapter 11	Semarang: A Brief Insight	109
Chapter 12	The Finishing Line	117
Chapter 13	An Insight into Patient Care	130
Chapter 14	Off Hospitals and Surgeries	141
Chapter 15	Experiencing PTSD	164
Chapter 16	Celebrating a Sense of Victory	176
Epilogue		201
References		202

Timeline and Glossary

1999 **Rectopexy, high anterior resection.** A type of colectomy that is the surgical removal of part of the bowel and anastomosis (joining) the two together.

2002 **Delorme procedure.** The removal of the outer layer of the prolapse bowel (instead of the whole prolapse) preserving the muscle layer which is then folded over like a concertina.

2004 **Laparoscopic rectopexy.** To correct and repair the rectal prolapse.

2010 **Ventral mesh rectopexy.** A procedure involving the suspension and fixation of the front of the rectum to the pelvic floor with a bio-dissolvable mesh.

2011 **Temporary loop ileostomy.** An opening at the terminal section of the small intestine allowing digestive waste to be discharged to a collection bag.

2013 **Total proctocolectomy with end ileostomy.** Surgery to remove all of the colon (larger intestine).

2017 **Laparotomy (two).** Removal of fifteen centimetres of the small bowel due to strangulation, acute haemorrhagic infarction and ischemic bowel.

2018 **Laparoscopic division of adhesions.** Release of adhesions (scar tissue)

Preface

In 2010 I made the decision to undergo stoma surgery after years of painful surgical procedures due to bowel disease. I had no idea where this would lead and how my life would change. Fortunately, I am now healthy and happy, a registered nurse and the mother of young Alexander. This is how it came about.

By 2019, with life progressing smoothly, I started to reflect on my seventeen years of ill health. This led to a compelling drive to tell of my experiences. My motivation was also fuelled by the encouraging responses I received at clinical workshop sessions where my peers and medical staff were keen to learn about ostomies in order to enhance the management of their patients.

Within the public arena, I discovered that many people were interested in learning about the ongoing life of a person living with an ostomy and other similar devices. Encouraging me also was the widespread belief that the will to fight on against all odds must be all encompassing, no matter the level of adversity. This positive interaction I received from audiences, underpinned by support I received from many other sources, convinced me that the role of an advocate could be rewarding and fulfilling.

As I developed my advocacy role and described the impacts and challenges in the life of an ostomate, I soon realised that I had much more to tell, and significantly many more people to reach. Hence my idea to write this book.

My intent is that it will serve as a general resource, and be of interest to those who care for and support the ostomate. More importantly, I hope that detailing the punishing phases of bowel illness, and showing how one can overcome most difficulties and survive, will give encouragement to others. It further shows that whatever the depth of adversity, there is always hope on the horizon: that resilience and perseverance must remain as critical elements in the journey to recovery.

In every sense, *Overcoming Fears and Tears: My Ostomy Story* is a reflection of enduring patience in searching for normality. I have cited examples of personal efforts as exemplary models of resilience. The book also encourages the patient's trust in the ability of the medical team to find appropriate solutions. Having full faith in the surgeon and others goes a long way towards winning the battle.

In this matter, I extend my heartfelt gratitude to my surgeon Dr John Lumley who tirelessly stood by me while I battled the illness. Without his skill and support, it is possible I would not be here to present this story.

As well, a special thanks to my gynaecologist Dr Ross Turner, who in the difficult times was a pillar of strength, particularly after life-threatening surgery and during so many emotional trials during my pregnancy.

And a special thank you to all of you who helped in many ways throughout the journey and who have influenced my life and achievements.

My heartfelt thanks to Dr Nadia Wright for her assistance in so many ways regarding the writing of this book. Her skills in advising on content, and her assistance in editing has been invaluable in the preparation of this manuscript.

A huge thank you to my husband Ben and members of the family for their continuous support as I battled seventeen years of adversity. Finally, a special thanks to my father, Bert Crathan, for the immense help and support in the writing of this book. Without his help this book would not have been possible.

Chapter 1

The Early Years

The biggest adventure you can take
is to live the life of your dreams.
— Oprah Winfrey

I was born in Melbourne in 1979 and named Kate Elizabeth. My parents, Ingrid and Bert, already had a son Benjamin and there was a second daughter after me: Jennifer. We are of mixed heritage, my father being Malaysian and my mother of Dutch ancestry. Our house was in Nicholas Street, a simple three-bedroom home in Ashburton, a suburb of Melbourne, which I remember fondly.

I attended Saint Michael's Primary School from Prep to Grade 6 and those years were normal in the sense that I participated in all aspects of school life. I was a competitive netball player and loved the sport. I was also an avid reader and spent many hours, especially during Melbourne's cold winters, with a book.

Growing up, I was mostly in good health apart from the usual childhood illnesses. From time to time, however, I remember the occasional stomach complaints, which would occur for no apparent reason. This resulted in my mother seeking advice from the doctor and a referral for assistance from child counsellors. The general opinion was that I may have been subject to some childhood stress, something hard to understand given that I was generally happy.

This was a long time ago, but my recollections are that following the usual physical medical examinations and counselling, there was no particular problem identified and life went on as usual. In hindsight, perhaps these episodes may have been the prelude to the problems that would surface later in life. Unfortunately, we will never know for certain.

I completed my Grade 6 primary education at Saint Michael's, and started my secondary schooling in 1992 at Avila College in Mount Waverley. This was an all-girls school not far from home.

In 1993 our family relocated to Queensland when my father secured a job in Brisbane.

In Brisbane I resumed my secondary schooling at Mt St Michael's College, a Catholic girls college located in the suburb of Ashgrove. The environment here was a complete contrast to my previous school. Ashgrove is an older suburb not far from the city centre; it is iconic with its period timber Queenslander-style houses, tin roofs and mango trees.

A feature of Mt St Michael's that stands out was the excellent care for the wellbeing of students. I am convinced that throughout the difficulties that occurred down the track, I know for a fact that I was able to *come through well* partly because of the influence of the school counsellors.

I can recall that in our discussions, the emphasis was always placed on the necessity to be resilient, no matter how difficult matters were. As I listened to this advice, I began to absorb this trait as a particular strength to nurture. I developed this as a useful tool as I went through life facing many of the problems and issues associated with the poor health that I was to endure. My sincere thanks to the school for the care and direction that was provided during the five years of learning at Mt St Michael's.

As I grew up, I loved school holidays and particularly the opportunity to travel, especially by air. I was always excited by plane travel, and I loved the atmosphere within the airports, particularly the constant buzz of activity. Sitting in the departure lounge, I would carefully observe all that was happening around me. When it was time to depart at the boarding gate, I was always in awe of the pilots and cabin crew, envious of all things about flying, and imagining how wonderful life must be for these people working in the industry.

I have no doubt that these experiences set me on a course towards a career in travel and hospitality, and as I continued my schooling, I was inevitably set on a trajectory that would allow me to work in the airline industry.

I completed my Year 12 studies in 1997 and in 1999 undertook a two-year course in hospitality management. I was feeling ready to take on the world and embark on a professional career. Importantly, I was still besotted with the hospitality industry incorporating travel and tourism, and my passion to work with the airlines as an in-flight stewardess.

Twelve months after graduation, and after working part-time in hospitality, I was secured a position at Virgin Airlines in its call centre in Brisbane. Although this was not ideal at the time, because I wanted to be an air stewardess, the opportunity did provide many insights into the broader picture of operations within the company. This then allowed me to gain a position later in ground staff.

The story that I will unfold in this book is about my health challenges starting at high school and extending through seventeen years of my life. In some detail I discuss the medical interventions being pursued right through to adulthood in an attempt to cure or fix the problem. As the period of my health crisis occurred over so many years, I have included the surgical events in the glossary as a reference of the events over the time of my illness.

As an impost on my life, I describe how this debilitating health condition impacted me so badly, while seeking to establish a successful career at Virgin Airlines. My story also relates to overcoming many obstacles in finally establishing a career in nursing, now a source of much satisfaction.

Most of all, this story is about the commitment required to seek a better quality of life, and the remedial and sometimes difficult actions that must be undertaken to achieve this crucial objective.

Chapter 2

Early Symptoms, Surgeries and Treatments

A great deal of our suffering comes from having too many thoughts. And, at the same time, the way we think is not sane. We are only concerned by our immediate satisfaction and forget to measure its long- term advantages and disadvantages, either for ourselves or for others. But such an attitude always goes against us in the end. There is no doubt that by changing our way of seeing things we could reduce our current difficulties and avoid creating new ones.

— Dalai Lama

My confronting bowel condition began at the age of sixteen while I was still at school.

I remember when this problem was first noticed. I was a healthy teenager, studying Year 11 at Mt St Michael's College in Brisbane. The first signs that a problem existed surfaced with the onset of crippling pains in my stomach and around the lower abdomen. Notably, this discomfort began to intensify as I moved from Year 11 through to Year 12, and by the end of Year 12 constant pain was the norm rather than exception.

Sometimes this pain was so intense that I was overcome with bouts of nausea, and succumbed to vomiting and severe diarrhoea.

These symptoms were a prelude to all that was soon to follow, manifesting itself into an ever-deteriorating condition I was going to endure for the next seventeen years. As the initial symptoms and potency intensified, it also started to have an impact on my lifestyle, forcing me to curb many of the activities that teenagers and young adults normally take for granted. This was a very distressing and sometimes awkward position for someone in my age group to cope with.

As an example, I recall the school formal when I was seventeen. This was the highlight of the school year and like my classmates I was looking forward to having a good time. However, there was a setback. Three days before the event, I started to feel unwell. To add to this distress was the fact that it was usual for these bouts of pain and discomfort to last for a few days. Thus, there was now a distinct possibility I would miss the formal.

Accepting that not attending would be a major disappointment, I steeled myself to overcome these barriers, and with the support and encouragement of my mother, I presented myself at the function.

So, even though I still had pain throughout the event, this was controllable, and coupled with a good stroke of luck, namely with the rare absence of toilet frequencies, I was able to get through that evening, and I actually enjoyed the formal.

The art of steeling is something I learned to adopt in response to each medical episode that occurred. This required managing thresholds of pain and as a tool to build barriers to overcome each bout of discomfort as far as possible. This deliberate action of switching off, involved turning the mind to more constructive and positive thoughts, and hence disassociation from the reality of what was actually happening inside the body. This was a helpful technique to control the pain while attending events.

It was the first of many lessons that I learned while overcoming pain and discomfort, a process that whenever possible I kept refining as the health problem became more difficult. In particular, this use of steeling became a useful ritual for daily survival, with varying degrees of success and failure, depending on the circumstances. Bearing in mind I was later employed for nearly thirteen years at Virgin Airlines, there were many instances where steeling was unsuccessful, a matter I will discuss in Chapter 3.

Like other parents, mine were no different, acknowledging the existence of some problem with the usual visits to doctors in an effort to find a diagnosis and a remedy. At this early stage, and in the opinion of the medicos, my youth was a major issue in the problem. They diagnosed that I was just a normal high school student experiencing the usual stresses of life. As a consequence, the doctors were comfortable in suggesting that the medical condition was not serious, stating that it was probably a mild case of irritable bowel syndrome (IBS), which was quite common.

Looking back all these years later, it is fair to say that this was a credible diagnosis as I was in the middle of my Year 12 studies and this period was often very stressful for students. Acknowledging all possible contributing factors, and some minor problems with my stomach and lower abdomen, it was considered that in time these symptoms would recede and life would be normal.

Supporting the initial diagnosis was the fact that over the following months my overall medical condition remained stable and was still manageable. Indeed, I was able to live quite comfortably on a day-to-day basis. I was confident in managing my problem, and in January 1997 I was able to travel overseas with my family to Malaysia and Singapore.

There were some difficult moments when I needed a quick exit in search of a toilet. In most cases this worked out satisfactorily. As far back as 1997 this was an early concern for me, but served as a good learning experience in managing toileting and hygiene when I later travelled to several developed and undeveloped countries. In particular, having this experience upfront was very important when travelling to Semarang in Indonesia in 2014, and living in a rural community as part of a training program.

From 1998 to 2000 my symptoms began to worsen with more and prolonged episodes of pain and discomfort. With the problem affecting work and studies, it became evident I needed to consult a specialist. Unless more assistance was provided, it would become increasingly difficult to function adequately in my daily life. After consulting my GP, and following a review of several specialists in this field, referrals to a colorectal surgeon and a gastroenterologist were recommended.

I was sent for a multitude of tests that included colonoscopies, colon transit studies, CT scans, a MRI, multiple blood tests and barium x-rays. The net result was that I was diagnosed with a prolapsed bowel, a condition normally associated with older persons, and certainly a rare condition for someone in my age group. It was so rare that the consultant had never treated this condition in a person of my age.

For those unfamiliar with this condition, a rectal prolapse is best described as the circumferential protrusion of the rectal wall through the anal canal. This condition is embarrassing and socially debilitating and causes pain, faecal incontinence, difficult evacuation, mucus discharge and bleeding. It was indeed consistent with all the symptoms that were constantly displayed starting from high school.

The colorectal surgeon recommended surgery. Receiving this diagnosis and the recommended medical intervention was a welcome relief. I thought: *Now that they know what is wrong, I can be fixed, and move on with a life free from pain, discomfort and, of course, be normal.*

So, in essence there was some feeling of euphoria because of the possibilities of an upside to life. Little did I know that I was actually at the starting blocks to a process that would later become the first of many corrective surgeries extending over many years.

The first surgery, which was the laparoscopic high anterior resection, was performed at the Wesley Hospital in Brisbane in 1999. This procedure was to remove a small section of the bowel where pockets had occurred and were deemed to be the source of pain and other symptoms. The prognosis was that once these offending areas were removed, the bowel itself, when rejoined, would operate normally. This operation was performed using keyhole surgery which was unintrusive and I was able to recover quite quickly.

As in this surgery, and others that followed, the recovery phase was an important time. I had the enhanced belief, not dissimilar to other patients undergoing similar treatments, that the corrective surgeries would identify the cause and rectify the problems identified. In every sense, a positive prognosis would be the least of my expectations. Naturally under these circumstances, the opportunity of being cured was foremost in my mind. In the recovery period I eagerly looked for every positive sign to indicate this was occurring.

Living with these expectations, I undertook a rigorous monitoring program to chart the progress of recovery. Certainly, in the early phases of recuperation there were some promising signs that indeed the corner had been turned. More encouragingly, some of the symptoms had disappeared while others had moderated to the extent that I was now feeling comfortable within myself that normality had indeed returned.

Then I hit the wall! About three weeks after the surgery there was a noticeable return to the previous problems consistent with the prolapsed bowel. With this change, the usual battles with constant pain were rekindled, and on the back of this, the accustomed poor cycle of health experienced prior to the surgery returned. To add to this disappointment, the frequencies of toilet visits were now back. I felt that nothing had been achieved.

The reality slowly unfolding was that this first corrective surgery was the start of the progression into a series of continuing medical procedures each one being a further intervening action in a vicious circle. In terms of providing a positive contribution, this first attempt, and the ongoing procedures, were nothing less than creating a downward spiral that could not be effectively controlled no matter the options and efforts attempted each time by the surgeons.

I am not being critical of the corrective surgeries that were performed. In fact, I remain very grateful to my medical team, and strongly believe that adopting corrective surgeries does provide an alternative option, especially in the case of difficult medical challenges. Importantly, corrective surgeries can also play a significant part in providing respite and a lot of hope. The latter is a critical factor in the support of patients seeking help.

In my case, and irrespective of the limited outcomes, I should emphasise that each time these surgeries were always necessary. On this basis, I always agreed with the surgeon's suggestions and recommendations.

I do feel that it was unfortunate the surgical interventions ended up mostly in limited outcomes because of the range of problems and complications. Despite the disappointments along the way there are no regrets, because if faced with a similar situation today, I would probably do it all over again.

Returning to square one after the first surgery was certainly extremely worrying. This need for a more effective solution was further compounded given the fact that I was now moving from casual work to full-time employment at Virgin Airlines. Clearly, I needed better assurance of more health stability because of the increasing demands of the job. Returning to the 'norm' was also depressing as I was working long hours, and the continuation of the previous cycle of pain and incontinency was now making life exceedingly more difficult. There was a desperate need to break the cycle of disruption. My recollection is that I was still positive, believing this was still just a hitch, and that a way around this problem would shortly be found.

Little did I know!

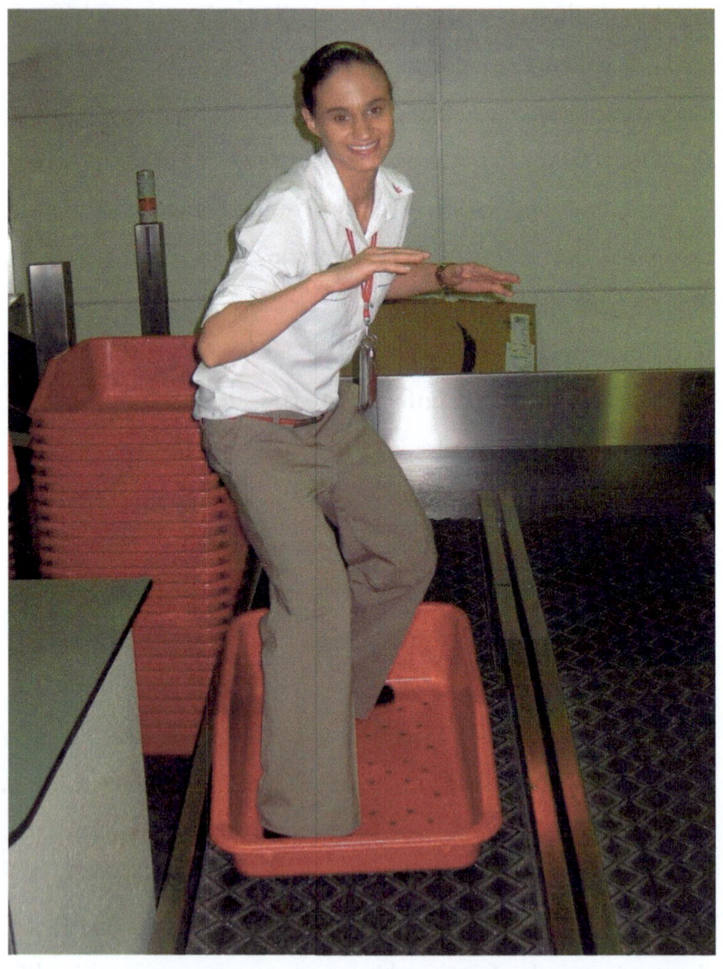

A lighter moment as Virgin Ground Crew

Chapter 3

The Airline Experiment

With the new day comes new strength and new thoughts.
Eleanor Roosevelt

It was not long after I had undergone the laparoscopic high anterior resection, described in the previous chapter, that I was offered another position in the airlines, moving from the call centre to ground staff. Again, I had missed out on the coveted air stewardess position, and the disappointment this time around was quite hard to accept. There was, however, a consolation prize. I had moved up the food chain, and I hoped that the next opportunity might yield the much sought-after job as a hostie.

Sometimes our disappointments can be further exacerbated by the knowledge that some of our colleagues and friends have been successful in gaining a position that is so much sought after by oneself. During the selection process, a good friend of mine was accepted as a flight stewardess. This was a bit heartbreaking and I wished that I could also join her as we worked so well together in the call centre. Nevertheless, I was happy for her.

Today she remains a close friend, and we continue to see each other at regular intervals even though neither of us works for Virgin Airlines.

There is a saying that there is a reason why certain events occurred, and this is so true in relation to my life. The medical challenges became progressively harder and in hindsight I can now accept that working as an airline stewardess would not have been sustainable, but that reality was far from my thoughts.

In November 2001, I began training. I was based at Brisbane Airport and enjoyed interesting and sometimes exciting times in a vibrant environment.

As a new employee, I underwent very comprehensive training as a consultant at the check-in desk, assisting in bookings, supporting customer needs and engaging with other operational areas within the system.

The training lasted four weeks and at the end of this period after being deemed competent enough for the tasks ahead, I received my uniform. A reward that immediately became my prized possession.

I could hardly wait to begin work in the real airline world doing exciting airline work, with an eagerness to embrace new challenges. Even now I can distinctly remember the first morning in this new position, and the excitement of walking into the bright lights and high energy of the departure area at Brisbane Airport, feeling cool in my new red Virgin uniform.

In my mind I had *arrived*.

By quickly utilising my experience of customer relations gained at the call centre, I was well into my stride. I worked an eight-hour shift, with the focus on delivering the ultimate travel experience. My personal presentation as an individual was expected to be exemplary. I was at all times required to deliver excellent service coupled with friendliness and patience at check-in, and at other locations in the airport.

My activities also extended to the boarding gate to complete arrival and departure procedures. Here the fun was to master the art of steering the aero bridge using mechanical controls to line up the equipment with the doors of the aircraft. While not difficult, it did require concentration and accuracy as the catchphrase was *don't bloody hit the plane.*

By 2004 I was now into a third surgery to fix the rectal prolapse, and although anticipating that this would bring a positive outcome, my condition in fact remained largely unchanged. Moreover, as time progressed it became obvious that the surgery was offering no respite, especially regarding increasing pain, discomfort and toilet frequencies. It was now evident that for me to work effectively, my situation had to be managed, so I could respond to the demands of many crucial tasks coming my way. At first, I used painkillers to support me through the day. Beyond this, and with no second option easily at hand, I then decided to use sheer willpower as a backstop. This was something quite difficult to undertake within a demanding environment.

To utilise sheer willpower in a work setting, the first challenge is to establish a mode of operating, or survival mode as I called it then. This was simply a tactic of using my mind to counteract the effects of the pain and discomfort, thus allowing me to function at some basic level. My particular approach was to operate within a bubble by focusing my mind away from the pain and discomfort whenever possible. Essentially this was no different to steeling, except performed at a much higher intensity and for longer periods. Looking back, I believe that the survival bubble technique served me quite well in the day-to-day activities, and through the different stages of the illness, surgeries and post-operative recoveries phases while I worked at Virgin Airlines. In particular, when the challenge was on, I was able to work effectively with a smile and friendliness – at least for some of the time. A word of caution, however! This idea may seem quite simple, but in practice it is quite difficult, and not necessarily suitable for everyone. It does depend on the circumstances of the existing medical condition.

Through all of this there was always in the recesses of my mind the underlying pressure of knowing that my health was continually heading downhill, and that at some time, perhaps sooner rather than later, more medical interventions were going to be required. True to form, these interventions did occur, amounting to a total of four surgeries when I worked at Virgin.

One of my confronting issues with working in the bubble was bowel inconsistency, resulting in constant visits to the toilet. There is no denying that this is an extremely difficult and very embarrassing situation for anyone, let alone someone involved in delivering customer service at a front desk. The most disturbing downside was the urgency at frequent and totally inconvenient times to vacate the workstation and go missing. This must have been disconcerting to my colleagues as well as the managers, because I usually returned each time looking and feeling completed wasted.

On reflection, notwithstanding the self-created bubble, I still find it difficult to comprehend how I managed to survive and retain my job in that extremely high-pressure environment. Survive I did! However, it came at a high physical and mental cost as at the end of each day I was totally exhausted, wondering what the next day would bring and how this cycle would be endured.

While the work was mostly enjoyable, the continuing health issues were destabilising with a slow build-up of pressure, as I knew that eventually the bubble would weaken, and even burst, resulting perhaps in catastrophic effects on work performance. Sitting on the edge filled me constantly with fear and despair, which often made me mentally distraught because of the fear of losing my job. These fears also extended to management, the unknown quantity being whether they fully comprehended my predicament, and were empathetic to my personal situation. Given that the focus of the organisation was on customer service, and with a worker being absent so often from the workstation, this could very well be viewed as unsatisfactory. It was difficult to see that management would think otherwise, and in my favour.

Then there were the fears that on very bad days I would not be able to last out the duration of my shift. Plus, there was the possibility of being overwhelmed by pain at a critical moment, and hence unable to cope with my tasks. All of this caused me much anxiety about my future career prospects in the organisation.

Amidst all the anxiety, I continued to soldier on, with 2005 being special, as in November that year I married Ben.

I had known Ben for some years as he also worked part-time in hospitality while he set about completing a qualification in graphic design. This was followed later with a stint in the Defence Force and a successful career in telecommunications.

Our marriage was held at the Capuchin Chapel, a little annex in St Stephen's Cathedral in Brisbane's Elizabeth Street. It was a family affair attended by relatives from interstate and many friends. It was a wonderful day for both of us as we embarked on our new life together after enjoying a memorable reception at the Marriott Hotel.

We rented a two-bedroom flat in Nundah, where we lived for the first two years of our marriage. Nundah is in a very convenient location as it is not far from the airport. It took me less than ten minutes to drive to the airport compared with the forty minutes normally spent commuting from The Gap where I had resided with my parents. It was a bonus, giving me more time to organise my daily routine.

Throughout my time at the airline, a factor that encouraged me was the support of some of my colleagues. In terms of management, it would be fair to say that on occasions I was given some leeway, although this was limited perhaps due to a lack of understanding of my health difficulties, or perhaps because of their own individual work pressures that took precedence over other matters.

Working at a check-in desk can be very demanding as the interaction with customers can vary markedly depending on the attitude of the individual being served. The following incident is an example of the support that I received from my workmates and their no-nonsense attitudes.

I recall a time when a customer vigorously challenged me over an overweight suitcase. Our training dictated that in this situation the traveller either voluntarily reduce the baggage weight or pay a surcharge. On this occasion the request resulted in abuse and, as the situation deteriorated, it also had an adverse impact across the area of operations, involving other travel consultants as well as passengers. My colleagues would never allow a member of the public to treat a co-worker in this manner, and before I knew it, a number of them had left their stations to quell this unjustified and abrasive dissent.

At the boarding gates my main tasks were to meet passengers on arrival and departure, and sometimes to address any queries from travellers. I enjoyed being at the boarding gates as a break from the check-in desk. However, even there I was regularly afflicted with the urgent need to use the toilets and sometimes just could not complete the job. In these instances, there were always others on duty who would respond by filling in for me and complete the task.

There were also times when the empathy of some staff members towards me was further demonstrated. During frantic peak holiday times some members of the team would give up their short breaks and relieve me, so that I could leave the desk as my bodily functions demanded.

I could not have asked for better colleagues to work with during my time at the airlines. To this very day I remain very thankful for the assistance they gave me. Their support helped keep me going throughout my thirteen years, and helped maintain my dreams of working in the airline industry. To all those who helped me, I can only say a huge thank you.

At the airlines I generally worked three eight-hour split shifts starting at 5.15 am, around midday or in the afternoon. The biggest issue affecting me was the intervening periods between shifts when I was never really well rested because of the lack of sleep. This remained a constant problem throughout my time with the company. Each night, getting enough sleep was a major issue because of ongoing discomfort, which I could temper somewhat by using medications.

Another debilitating problem outside of constant pain was incontinence requiring frequent visits to the toilet during the night. This kept me awake regularly and was terribly disruptive to sleep patterns resulting in insufficient rest. This became more testing with early morning shifts. I had to get out of bed by 3.30 am to begin the 5.15 am shift. I got up feeling absolutely fatigued, and from one work cycle to the next this had a compounding negative effect. It was a continuous pattern of insufficient sleep followed by little or no recovery from the efforts of the previous day.

Clearly in the current situation, any respite, however short, was always very welcome. So, I looked forward to the off-duty days and the chance to catch up on much-needed rest and recovery. Annual holidays, public holidays and any scheduled time-off were highly sought throughout this period. To best describe my lifestyle over the greater part of thirteen years was the absence of any social life.

In my working life today as a nurse, I still engage in shift work of a similar magnitude, but I manage this with little difficulty largely because of the improvements to my health.

I persisted with my ambition to secure a position as cabin crew, and in 2009 when a temporary position became available in Airport Movement Co-ordination or AMCO, I applied. This was hands-on activity involving direct communications with the pilots of an aircraft while in-flight. Basically, I had to provide information in relation to fuel loads and the fuel requirements of each aircraft depending on its daily travel schedules and routes flown.

I viewed this job as a chance of gaining added experience and knowledge about aircraft operations and procedures through interactions with the cockpit. I felt that it would also enhance my chances in securing a position as cabin crew.

I was successful in my application and I was reassigned to the temporary position at AMCO. I was excited at the prospect of engaging in a new learning experience, at a new workstation, with a new set of work mates. It was all looking good.

Initially this work was quite rewarding, however, in time the tasks started to become quite repetitive, sometimes tedious and falling short of my expectations. There was one positive element of this position in that it afforded me better management of the prevailing medical difficulties. There was no direct contact with the public, and therefore generally less concern about regularly vacating the workstation to visit the toilet. This was indeed a bonus, and certainly less stressful.

Overall, toilet frequencies and episodes of pain still posed a problem, and the reality that crucial tasks, if imperfectly performed, could directly impact air safety. So, there was still the retention of a high level of stress and anxiety to do it right. This required working hard at absorbing the personal health discomforts while performing at the highest level possible.

The post at AMCO was for six months, and at its conclusion there was some relief in returning to the ground staff position. In hindsight, while this assignment did not realise many of the perceived expectations, and did not bring me any closer to achieving the coveted cabin crew position, I acquired additional skills and made new friends.

In all I spent thirteen years at Virgin, from 2000 to 2013. This allowed me to realise some of my childhood dreams in the fabulous world of air travel.

Chapter 4

The Desperate Search for a Breakthrough

Life is not a matter of holding good cards,
but of playing a poor hand well.
— Robert Louis Stevenson

In 2001 when I was promoted from the call centre in Brisbane Airport to work as ground staff, I also began the search for other medical options to address my health problems. At this time, finding new solutions were indeed a priority, as it was now two years since the initial unsuccessful first surgery, and sadly nothing had improved. The need for respite was urgently required, firstly to improve the quality of life, and then to be medically fit to manage the complexities associated with having to work in a demanding and complex environment.

This chapter provides a more detailed account of the time spent in seeking a medical breakthrough while still working at Virgin. It reflects the remedial actions and the associated surgical interventions that were undertaken over a long period of thirteen years. This search was urgently needed because of the concern that my physical condition was worsening, and with it, increasing restrictions were being cumulatively imposed on me.

Not long after the first surgery, as my medical condition started to deteriorate, and the situation became somewhat more desperate, I consulted my surgeon. The usual tests were undertaken and my worst fears realised when it was confirmed that in the last two years another prolapse had developed. He recommended further surgery as the only viable option to rectify the problem.

On the basis that the pervious attempt to repair the prolapse was unsuccessful, an alternative procedure was recommended. The proposal was essentially to hitch the bowel up to keep it in place. The clinical rationale here is that by hitching the organ upright it would in turn stabilise in a secured position, and by doing so would prevent another prolapse occurring. This is known as a Delorme's procedure.

I was now just 22 and completely devastated by the notion that I was off again to face a second attempt at colorectal corrective keyhole surgery.

After researching the relevant literature on this procedure, I remained quite confident of a good result. I was also buoyed by the fact that as the condition does not readily occur in people of my age, the chances of being fully rectified were high. Filled with hope, although there were still bucket loads of apprehension, I decided to have another go, and presented myself at The Wesley Hospital for the second shot at bowel surgery.

At post-surgery, my hopes were again lifted when my surgeon confirmed that the operation went well, and he was hopeful about achieving a good result this time around. Very encouraged by the news, I progressed through the normal recuperation stages always looking in anticipation for any changes or signs that would indicate a positive advancement, particularly to changes in the digestive tract. The prevailing feelings were somewhat of a rollercoaster ride with hopes rising and falling, and the propensity to grasp at any sign, real and sometimes even illusionary, that suggested that finally something was working right, and a full recovery was in sight.

In hindsight, I guess I must be a glutton for punishment, as over the course of all the procedures I always kept anticipating that *this time* it was going to work, and directed my psyche towards a positive result. Fortunately, over the period of four surgeries I learned to temper these feelings by adjusting my mindset towards a position of avoiding overly optimistic outcomes, and steer clear of the resultant despair.

In this second attempt, the initial results again showed early promise. However, towards the end of the recovery period the symptoms common in the past few years re-emerged. So, what initially looked like the chance of a respite was actually a false dawn. In reality, the constant pain followed by toilet frequencies returned to its usual intensity. I was back to my normal, and hence, square one.

My response after this second failure was: *Where do I go from here?* I initially felt that to adopt the view that there was nowhere to go, would be to capitulate, a position I refused to accept. So, I again began to research alternatives or options, delving into books, magazines, the internet, and having discussions with people knowledgeable in this area. Most of the literature and advice was from medical experts who could provide a professional opinion, or from information drawn from persons with the experience of living with a similar type of medical condition.

The idea behind seeking alternative treatments was centred on the possibility that perhaps during my diagnoses something had been missed. If this was the case, then alternative treatments or approaches might provide some direction for an ultimate solution to the problem. I again consulted with my medical advisors, and by mutual agreement, I was off meeting with other specialists in an attempt to find different solutions. Although it remained unclear why the surgeries had been unsuccessful, the decision to try other strategies was worth the effort and one I fully supported.

The new strategy was to return to some basics using supplementary specialists including a dietitian and a physiotherapist. The choice of a dietitian was obvious. Proper dieting, avoiding certain foods and focusing on others more suitable would enhance and improve the workings of the digestive system. The ultimate intent was that if the diet complemented the performance of the digestive track, this could perhaps work in tandem with the recent surgery, and hence aid in the healing process.

Thus, I followed the suggested food regime and established eating patterns that would assist digestion. Diligently I kept on this path for a period of some six months, but it became clear that this was not going to be the solution to the problem. All the familiar symptoms continued to persist. In fact, there were no changes to the toilet frequencies. I had again reached an impasse in finding a solution.

A physiotherapist was proposed on the basis that specific exercises directed at the bowel area and the digestive system might improve the function of the muscles so they would settle into a rhythm and perform in the normal manner. Similar to the dieting option, it was considered that this strategy of working in tandem with the recent surgery might bear some positive results. I thus attended regular sessions with a physiotherapist for some three months. The exercises were very intense and thorough, directed at stimulating a change in the mechanics controlling the muscles associated with the bowel.

Being always hopeful, I persisted with this therapy, seeking the breakthrough that I so desperately wanted, and one that never came. Sadly again, there was little improvement for all my efforts. There was no observable progress, and importantly, except for a brief period of limited relief, all the symptoms remained. I was back to square one!

Let me emphasise that I have a high opinion of specialists such as physiotherapists, masseurs and dietitians, as they provide a value-added service and support as members of the wider medical community. Throughout my personal battles these practitioners were constantly available to provide pain relief and general support. I have found them and their commitment exemplary. Therefore, in the years involving the surgeries I had no hesitation in using these services as a source of medical relief. Today, as appropriate, I still draw on them for various forms of support.

That these specialists were unable to successfully intervene and assist me in the years spent looking for a resolution is perhaps because my medical condition was clearly unique and complicated.

In many ways it defied all the usual norms associated with, and generally known about, the condition. The medical responses displayed after the surgeries also seemed to baffle the surgeons, so it must have been equally difficult and challenging for the physiotherapists, dietitians and others to achieve a more conclusive result.

So, while every effort was made by the therapists, resulting in little change, it was now time to return to the familiar route of more consultations with the doctors and again explore additional medical alternatives or options.

This was indeed a very pressing time as it was 2004 and I was well and truly entrenched as a member of ground staff at Virgin Airlines. It was clear that it would be very difficult to develop my career there unless a suitable solution to my problem could be found.

So, with two surgeries down and no success, the medicos were again approached. This time I emphasised the dire situation currently at work, and begged for more assistance so that I could function just a little better. I repeated that any efforts in making my life less of a misery would be a bonus, and I implored the medicos to reduce the persistent pain and discomfort, and as much as possible help me control the toilet frequencies.

It was another *here we go again,* as after consultations and reviews of the information based on the previous surgeries, it was suggested that another procedure be considered using a different technique. This time the proposal was to perform a laparoscopic rectopexy, a different procedure, and one also used to repair a rectal prolapse. Here the rectum is restored to its normal position in the pelvis, so that it no longer protrudes through the anus. Usually, stitches are used to secure the rectum, together with a mesh. At this time, laparoscopic rectopexy was used by many pelvic floor surgeons because of the good results, particularly in improving or repairing the functionality of the rectum.

In the light of the previous failures, there was obviously still much concern about the procedure, and the likelihood of its success. As well, there were also problems about the time I would be away from work. I had already been on sick leave on a number of occasions, and the capacity for my employer to grant further leave was now almost stretched to its limits.

In the end there was little choice but to try again. I was admitted to The Wesley Hospital for this surgery to be performed by the primary surgeon looking after me.

This time around there was a little more confidence; this being buoyed by the research I had undertaken confirming a high rate of success of a laparoscopic rectopexy. My expectations of a resolution were therefore also high. Not trying to be over optimistic, I did feel that there was sufficient evidence for a good chance of success. I hoped this attempt would at the very least provide some marginal improvements to my condition, and with it a discernible reduction in pain and discomfort. Even partial success would provide me with better control of my day-to-day activities.

Outside the work environment, I felt that any improvement, however small, would be an important ingredient in enhancing my overall quality of life, for up to this point it was already quite poor and getting worse.

Moving into my third bowel operation in about three years, it was reasonable to conclude that a positive outcome was on the cards. The apparent success of this technique, and my confidence in the knowledge and skill of the medical team, led me to believe I could not possibly lose. Or so, I thought. Alas, the answer was again an emphatic *No!*

This was again another major disappointment to overcome, because the pain and discomfort returned with *full vengeance.* The word 'vengeance' is used to describe the situation because on some days the pain was in regular patterns that was more intense and harder to manage than before. More discouraging was the fact that this was different from the previous surgeries in that the pain and discomfort returned within a much shorter time.

Another backward step resulting from the laparoscopic rectopexy surgery was its impact on my toilet frequency. Most disconcertingly, I could no longer eat a full meal without rapidly having to dash to the nearest bathroom. With these increased frequencies there was also blood loss due to an ulcer in the rectum. This resulted in anaemia. I became easily exhausted, and together with all the previous symptoms, the poor sleep patterns that were constantly being experienced, continued. To say at this juncture that my daily struggles had now increased four-fold was clearly an understatement.

The hardest part to tolerate with the regression in my health was the capacity to attain my work performance benchmarks. They became a much bigger challenge to achieve. So, in this evolving scenario, the interplay of forces between the medical distress and the capacity to perform normal tasks became a tight balancing act and one that was almost impossible to sustain over any period of time.

Once again, there was nowhere else to go, and as the days and weeks progressed, I lost my enthusiasm and willingness to fight on. I was aware that if the situation referred to earlier as the *full vengeance* persisted, there would be an urgent need for further medical support. It was back to the doctors as usual, and as an immediate countermeasure, painkillers were prescribed. Thus, within a short time following the third surgery, I was increasingly dependent on heavy strength painkillers as the alternative treatment.

With the failure of the third attempt at corrective surgery and the situation deteriorating, coping with daily life was now stretched to the limit, with my emotional state in total freefall. In progressing downwards, I now had distinct feelings of depression and this became problematic. In hindsight, I now believe that this was likely a response to self-pity, and was the first of a number of lessons to learn when a person faced with such trying circumstances lets his or her guard down.

Letting one's guard down and allowing despair to become the driver is a terrible position. I began to weigh myself down asking: *Why has this occurred to me? Why am I being robbed of the right to a normal existence like everyone else around me?* Looking back, I can somehow understand my reactions at the time because I was seemingly stuck in a revolving door with nowhere to go.

Engaging in self-pity is difficult to avoid when trying to live a normal lifestyle like going to work, travelling and socialising without having to combat pain, discomfort and the embarrassing toilet frequencies. This is never easy even when utilising coping mechanisms such as personal resilience and strength of conviction that a cure was just around the corner. As I tried desperately to move positively forward, these coping tools were never good enough. Gradually, the poor quality of life began to overwhelm me emotionally to the point where there was a definite downhill trajectory, which was very difficult to reverse despite my efforts.

My advice to others caught in a similar position is to always remember that despite the setbacks there are options available to counter what is seemingly a hopeless situation. While a cure is the ultimate goal, it may in many instances be some distance away, and therefore finding different methods to counter setbacks is a way of moving forward. In the light of my experience, I fully support the approach of pushing hard against the tide as continued perseverance will ultimately bring many of the rewards desired. I firmly believe this is a good strategy, and one that was reaffirmed when I encountered other ostomates including Canadian Jessica Grossman, whom I will discuss in a later chapter, as someone who has successfully pushed hard against the tide.

I must admit to being slow off the mark in pushing against the tide, but from experience gained it surely does work. So, take it on and you will avoid the unnecessary downhill slide that I experienced for a short period of time, before realising the folly of my ways.

So, after three disappointing operations there was little upside left but to consider the *what next?* strategy.

There were basically three possible courses of action available.

Firstly, there was the need to look at the situation objectively and accept the reality that until a remedy was found, there was no option but to live and endure the predicament on a daily basis as best I could. Secondly, as a matter of priority, there was the urgency to address the added complication of anaemia due to frequent blood loss, and that there was the necessary medical support in place. If left unchecked it could be life threatening. As the last step, there was still the need to search for other alternative medical options, and to explore these with the medical team.

In respect to the anaemia, my GP was consulted and prescribed supplements such as iron tablets and a recommended diet of particular vegetables to replenish iron. Indeed, while the blood loss persisted consistent with the continued toilet frequencies, these remedies greatly helped to manage the situation, and assisted in making me feel less exhausted, and therefore offered a welcome short-term reprieve.

As for managing daily life, it is important to be realistic. There are many confronting challenges and indeed very difficult tasks to undertake on an ongoing basis. I am limited in my advice, as each person is faced with different circumstances, and whatever is said here about my actions at the time does not come with any guarantees that it would apply to someone else. My advice here is to keep pressing head-on despite the days of despair and distress, and be diligent in working through all the avenues available to achieve an acceptable solution.

Turning to my medical team for more ideas and pressing for solutions and answers to particular issues became unnerving. Their responses suggested that they were quickly running out of ideas. Never willing to give up, I desperately searched the internet and other medical resources for other viable solutions. In doing so I came across a professor of colorectal surgery operating out of Melbourne. In reviewing his work, I felt quite enthusiastic, as it appeared that this specialist could perhaps offer an alternative solution that may assist. Specifically, the technique on offer was called a 'J Pouch'. In broad terms this hitches the bowel in a shape of the letter J, which in theory would better manage movement through the bowel. I thought that if movement through the bowel was better managed, then this would in turn control toilet frequency and contain the pain.

In my keenness to try anything, my mother and I travelled to Melbourne for a face-to-face consultation. The surgeon read all my clinical notes from previous treatments and surgeries. He then concluded that he could not guarantee a satisfactory outcome in any surgery that he undertook. It was clear that the J Pouch was not necessarily an alternative for me at all. With this rebuff, it is very difficult to describe my feelings of despondency as we flew back that same day to Brisbane, especially knowing that now there seemed less hope for a medical resolution that was desperately needed.

It was now 2009. Following the disappointment of Melbourne, and also knowing that the local medicos had become reluctant to engage in any further attempts at surgery or other interventions, I still refused to give up. I arranged another meeting with my specialist medical team. The best they could recommend was to establish a holding patten while engaging in a series of routine tests to look for changes that may have occurred. Broadly, the idea behind these tests was to establish and identify some definitive indicators that would support another way forward. It was clearly a safety-first approach given all the previous setbacks from the earlier attempts.

As I waited and waded through the tests it was hard to believe my eyes when the results came through. I had now developed another prolapse. To complicate matters further was the added problem of a medical condition known as a pelvic floor drop.

To explain this briefly, the pelvic floor is made up of a group of muscles and ligaments that support the bladder, uterus and bowel. When the pelvic floor is strong, it supports the pelvic organs to prevent problems such as incontinence and the involuntary loss of urine and faeces. In a normal pelvic floor, support is provided to the bowel and prevents a prolapse from occurring. However, when the pelvic floor drops a person suffering this condition is now subject to further degradation of the already poor digestive and bowel functions, and hence moving into more difficult territory.

With this new development, I was told that immediate surgery was required. If the procedure was not quickly performed it would lead to further deterioration of the prolapse, in turn resulting in increased frequency of incontinence. Incontinence was the main problem here, because increased frequency would not only result in more pain, but importantly, increased blood loss, a condition that was already adversely affecting me. As previously mentioned, the concern about this increased blood loss was its potential to be life-threatening, and the effective measure was urgent surgical intervention because of the risk involved. While the information initially came as somewhat of a shock, I was resigned to the fact that there was little choice but to succumb to a fourth operation. The situation was beyond a quality-of-life issue and needed to be resolved quickly.

The fourth major bowel operation was a procedure called a laparoscopic ventral mesh rectopexy (LVMR), a variation of the previous surgery undertaken a few months earlier. This time the procedure included the insertion of a mesh, and basically the LVMR was intended to straighten and attach the rectum back into its normal position within the pelvis. The rectum would be then kept in this position using the mesh. The mesh itself is made from synthetic material, basically plastic similar to nylon, and it is stitched to the front of the rectum and secured to the sacrum, or lower backbone. The purpose of the procedure is to pull the bowel up out of the pelvis and prevent it from telescoping down, thereby restoring the organ to its normal anatomical position.

I was admitted to the Holy Spirit Northside Private Hospital, teetering on the edge of despair and trying desperately to shut down all the voices in my head while undergoing the accustomed pre-operative procedures. I recollect when awakening in the recovery ward that I had undergone a fairly long surgical procedure.

This time the physical process of recovery was very different as I started to struggle with food intake brought on by a loss of appetite. Before I became fully aware, my weight plummeted, adding further concern to myself and the medical team. Also, with this surgery there was a much longer recuperative period because of my poor state of mind, generally poor bodily health, coupled with the added complexity of the procedure. This longer recuperative period meant that I could not return to work, which was very disconcerting as I had taken so much sick leave to address all the recurring health problems.

Unfortunately, this fourth attempt, resulted in no tangible success. There was no change to the condition and all the usual symptoms of discomfort persisted. My experience now told me that there were still other hurdles to overcome. I needed to reassess the situation and combat any negative responses or else fall prey to a state of despair and depression.

In reviewing my medical history, it can appear that bowel surgeries are tricky procedures with much potential for yielding poor results for the patient. Let me say unequivocally, that this is definitely not the case. It is very unlikely that people stricken with a bowel disease and other digestive problems will have a similar level of complications requiring the need to undergo the number of surgeries that I was confronted with. In hindsight, it is clear that my experience suggests an unusual case. Under normal circumstances these procedures are usually followed by good or very acceptable outcomes for the patient. These surgeries are aimed at remedial action, and the surgeons will usually find the answer and successfully resolve the problem. Therefore, my advice to anyone facing bowel surgeries is to remain strong and be emboldened with a sense of hope built around an unswerving belief that your medical specialists *would nail it this time around.*

It was time to reboot and the best recourse was to turn to the bigger picture, and to be objective, knowing that I was only thirty-one years old with time on my side. My youth, coupled with the usual expectations of persons my age, made me resolve to fight back hard, and to pursue the belief that an answer is always around the corner.

In the meantime, I remained conscious of the fact that in time my bodily health would continue to decline, unless appropriate measures were undertaken to redress this situation. I remained committed to making calculated and appropriate decisions. A major part of this was a promise to myself to never find a reason to relent, and allow nature take its course. I knew full well that this pathway would lead to a quality of life and a future not worth considering.

In confronting each setback, I was increasingly determined to believe in my medical team. In my opinion, the primary surgeon responsible for my care is second to none, and clearly to retreat from his commitment at that critical time, while he was in every way still in my corner, would not make any sense. Thinking where I am now, and living my life in a happy and resourceful manner, it is evident that the trust I placed in the medicos was well founded. I am here and well, largely because of the efforts of the team and the surgeon, their expert medical knowledge, and their empathy displayed throughout my struggles.

The important message is to never give up because there will be light at the end of the tunnel. Gaining a chance to experience any improvement in one's quality of life is always a welcome bonus. One must always be prepared to accept and consider all options and solutions, even though the ultimate choice in some instances may not be the best one you could wish for. The support and encouragement of family becomes crucial in this phase of the journey, being a stabilising influence when one is constantly on edge. I found that seeking input and support from my family in the broader consultative process with surgeons became immensely valuable, particularly when difficult decisions were to be made.

Meanwhile, more tests were ordered in the hope that something might be discovered to indicate another approach to treat the problem, and in a best-case scenario even find a cure. Mostly these tests were a repeat of the ones undertaken when the problem was first presented to the medicos. They were to discover if there were any significant changes to the digestive system that had occurred over time, and importantly, if there were any issues of concern that needed immediate action.

In October 2011, there came a major blow to my confidence. It was discovered after further tests that there had been a major change to the mechanics of the bowel. Results revealed that a significantly diminished holding capacity had now developed, meaning that the current incontinences and toilet frequencies would be on the increase. Perhaps due to my past experiences I should have expected this outcome, as I distinctly remember at this time consistently experiencing more pain coupled with an increasing frequency in toilet usage. In my mind I knew that something additional was amiss, and in my effort to dodge the bullet, I sought to deflect any negative thoughts by thinking it was nothing serious.

As a result of this finding, the surgeon ordered further investigations, which revealed the beginning of an intussusception. This is best described as the bowel folding itself into a telescope, with the folding having the potential to block the bowel and its blood supply causing further damage to the organ. To the best of my knowledge and experience, this was just another prolapse, but certainly of a different kind.

So, there it was, with the first prolapse surgery in 1999 and all the remedial action, and now twelve years on with another prolapse! Distressingly, over all these years there was little or no progress made. I cannot succinctly describe my emotions, but in simple terms it was like being torn apart, knowing I was back at square one after all the effort, disappointments and pain.

As always, it was again time to take some control of the situation. It was now clear that the upward trajectory in the battle for wellness was going to be an even steeper curve. At that moment I felt almost justified in thinking that the chances of any recovery were becoming more remote and distant, given that every procedure and surgical technique had been tried, and nothing positive had materialised. After working through my total despair at the onset of this awful news, I met with the primary surgeon, who acknowledged that while everything had been tried, the issues and symptoms relating to the bowel continued to persist. He indicated that there was little else to offer beyond further surgery. There was only one option left: to undergo a temporary loop ileostomy.

This is a procedure designed to disconnect the bowel at the point where the small bowel and the large bowel meet, thus allowing for all waste produced by the body to be discharged directly from the small intestine to a bag attached to the body. The objective is that this temporary measure will allow the large bowel to rest, and that the prolonged rest would heal the organ and then allow it to function normally. This was the medical rationale given by the doctors, and although there were many reservations, there was also a need to give this option serious consideration.

In terms of personal concerns, the most unthinkable and off-putting is having a waste bag attached to the body. I regarded this as an unnatural state of existence, and a disbelief that anyone can live normally with such an impediment. It must be said that for a person facing this possibility for the first time, it is not unusual to react with almost pure fear, driven by one's perceived stigmas associated with a waste bag.

For those who have already faced this dilemma, I am certain you will understand my feelings.

So, the most critical moment in my life arrived at the age of thirty-one. I was facing a life-changing situation in deciding to undertake such a procedure. Processing the potential repercussions of this decision, especially when visualising what it would look like in reality, caused me much emotion and fear. Those fears were beyond anything that can easily be described.

Clearly for a person to have a waste bag is certainly very confronting because of the reality of the situation, no matter from which angle this is viewed. This abnormality can be very difficult for anyone facing this future, particularly about the negative impacts of the device, and how to live with it.

In living with this device, this issue about stigmas is not as confronting as it may seem, as it is widely known that many people have bags attached to their bodies, most commonly after bowel cancer surgery. In the main, those in contact with someone who has a bag are very understanding and sympathetic towards the person. A clear reflection of the prevailing human spirit.

Anecdotally, however, there is another worrying side to this. Some individuals can appear to act in a distant manner towards a person with an ileostomy or colostomy, maybe because of non-acceptance or reasons such as a lack of understanding. Broadly described as rejection on the grounds of a prevailing social stigma associated with a stoma was the fear that I was most concerned about.

Adding to this dilemma, I had no idea how to manage work at the airlines. Having a waste bag would entail emptying, cleaning and attending to other matters relating to a stoma. This would create a significant change to my lifestyle and work patterns. Ahead of me lay a much different world with the possibilities of a complex future, filled with many uncertainties.

This was now the crossroad! I would have to give serious consideration and consent to a medical procedure which, from my personal perspective, seemed extremely radical. This required some very hard thinking, much convincing and justification from the doctors, and also support and reassurance from family members.

I began this chapter seeking a breakthrough, and although the current proposition was not an attractive alternative, it was still a matter, however unappealing, that had to be objectively considered. The consequences of dismissing this option could effectively mean confinement to living an ongoing difficult life. On the other side of the ledger, the consequences of having the procedure posed many difficult questions, and I was left to ponder all possible scenarios, knowing that a difficult decision was just around the corner.

Chapter 5

Hard Decisions

You gain strength, courage and confidence by every experience in which you really stop to look fear in the face … You must do the things which you think you cannot do.

— Eleanor Roosevelt

So, I was now faced with this question: *How does a young woman at the age of 31 come to terms with the idea of having a stoma?* Then there was the corresponding issue constantly at play in the back of my mind. *How am I going to walk around with a bag attached to my body collecting my waste, an intrusive and offensive appendage.*

In this sense, the idea of a stoma instantly generated added fears about perceptions of a woman with a waste disposal bag attached to her body. Consequently, my first response was that it was a bridge too far for the mind to objectively grapple with. A classic response was to visualise the scene when walking around with this intrusive appendage to the body, and how I was going to hide it. This was constantly my concern due to the prevailing view that this situation happens to older people, which is a misplaced belief that I later came to realise.

This was the confronting reality when the surgeon informed me that no other alternatives were available to alleviate the problem. More confronting was that this was a last-ditch effort to stem any further deterioration in my health.

To be honest, up to this point there were never any thoughts that in the course of my illness, a waste bag attached to my body would be needed. In fact, never at any time was there the feeling that the situation would be serious and life threatening enough to warrant going down this path, until this moment of truth arrived.

The surgeon was forthright, pointing out that everything possible had now been attempted without success. He went on to say he was very worried at my worsening condition. There were no other viable options. In reality, the only positive to take away from a long-term prognosis was his recommendation that the ileostomy be considered as a temporary fixture. Should the bowel repair itself there was still a good chance for a normal life. Most troubling in discussing this option was the revelation that without this surgery there was a possibility I would not live beyond the age of forty. The goalposts had indeed shifted! It was now not just a question of mitigating the downside effects of a difficult anatomical bowel, but also one of long-term survival.

To put it simply, I was terrified. I cried for weeks, grappling with fears of the unknown including the fact that while entrenched in the airlines, I was barely surviving, and therefore fearful of what the future would hold.

In a small way, however, one major reason for having an ileostomy that did provide some comfort was the data that I had gathered when researching the procedure. It confirmed a temporary ileostomy could be a viable option for me. Knowing also that the choice of a temporary or permanent stoma were decisions to be made further down the track placated me somewhat, and I was prepared to accept the advice of the surgeon and proceed with the surgery.

In visualising life as an ostomate a major issue was the inevitable question of fashion and dress sense. Let me describe myself. I am 145 centimetres tall and weigh forty-seven kilograms. Being partly of Asian descent, I have a small frame and fit comfortably into shapely clothes; the best example is the sarong kebaya worn by the female cabin crew on Singapore Airlines, who are known affectionately as the Singapore Girls. I have a sarong kebaya and believe I could easily pass as one of the Singapore Girls.

Given my physical appearance, there was a major concern about the clothes I would have to wear, and with it, the inevitable restriction in the choice of dress to hide the stoma. A whole new wardrobe would be required, doing away with the style of clothes that were up to this point a key part of my persona.

Another area of concern was the continuing perceived stigma that exists in some parts of society when confronted by a person with a waste bag. In particular, not having a clear picture of the reactions of people when in contact with an ostomate was a challenging thought, and increasingly became very disconcerting. Before my illness, my limited understanding of persons with waste bags were those usually suffering serious bowel conditions, and had bags attached to their bodies after surgery. In my youth it was easy to be indifferent and dismissive of this issue, perhaps even to the point of being a little bit squeamish around people with colostomy bags. Therefore, in my developing mindset, there were strong concerns and fears about the reactions of friends and workmates. I was terrified that they would have similar reactions in my presence.

In respect to the workplace, this level of uncertainty continued to build, particularly when considering the practicalities of working with a bag, and the effects this would have on my daily performance. I worried about interactions with my colleagues, and also had thoughts of both parties being embarrassed about my new medical condition. *Was my working life now going to be problematic?*

The one positive factor I was able to cling to was the fact that previously I was able to cope with my workmates. So, at least there was this positive feeling coupled with some good measure of hope that the status quo would resume.

Most worrisome was the constant threat of accidents from leakages, or total failure of the bag, which can occur at the most inappropriate of times. Much worse was the horrifying thought of such an incident occurring while attending to a customer at the check-in desk. Adding to this was also the fear that a failure of the system could occur on public transport, in a bus or a train, or dare I say it, on a plane.

Then of course there was the question of maintenance, which requires going to the toilet to empty the accumulated waste. There were also the issues associated with proper sanitary practices, a matter to be acutely aware of in the choice to live with an ileostomy.

Apart from the concerns of my workmates and friends,

more worrying was the impact that a stoma would have on my husband. Ben and I were married two years earlier, and prior to our marriage he was fully aware of the medical problems I was enduring, considering it as part of the challenges of life. In all this time he was always supportive, however, even with the benefit of hindsight, it would be reasonable to say that it was unlikely he would have envisaged I would be fitted with a stoma as a long-term proposition.

While waiting for the inevitable change in lifestyle and the adjustments that were coming, I will take some time here to pay tribute to my husband. From the outset Ben was a rock by my side over the years living with all the surgical interventions, never wavering, and staying optimistic that somehow a solution would be found; ultimately being fully convinced that normality would eventually prevail.

My relationship with Ben had started not long before I underwent some of the early corrective surgeries and he invariably became part of the many disappointments that followed each unsuccessful attempt at remediation. I can also recall that each time the surgery failed, Ben, like myself, would also become devastated; however, through all this he was quick to recover from the disappointments, always managing a positive attitude that success was attainable. This approach became infectious, and assisted in the building of my strength to keep pursuing different avenues in search of a cure. It was this support and encouragement that finally convinced me to make the decision to accept the ileostomy as the best deal available.

I still find it difficult to truly comprehend how Ben must

have felt through all those years of multiple surgeries with little to show for the efforts involved. To put this into its proper perspective, Ben was thirty-five years old at the time of the impending stoma operation and clearly a young male in the prime of this life. Therefore, looking at the situation from his position, it must have been very difficult for a young husband when faced with all the unpalatable outcomes that could be on offer. It is hard to rationalise his confrontation with reality, that he would have a young wife who would be different from others, as now the woman he has married would have a bag as her waste disposal unit. This must have been an added burden to carry. He had already witnessed so many failures, and given the track record of the past, his belief this situation could likely continue, even with this recommended procedure, was a reasonable assumption. Added to this were the challenges of living a normal existence as a married couple, and our intimate relationship. This included the confronting question of having children, which must have been playing on his mind, because he was very much looking forward to being a father.

Through all this, Ben never wavered in believing that this current proposition was somewhere towards a viable solution and in the best interests of both of us. Being pragmatic, he believed that irrespective of the personal hurdles, and no matter what transpired, it would work out, because adjustments to life can always be made. His conviction at the time was much stronger than mine, and certainly an expression of his resilience. In both our minds the ileostomy was a massive game changer, and throughout this difficult period he took it fully in his stride, displaying strength of character, and transferring some of this to me as I approached the time of reckoning.

Besides my husband, the support of my family when I was struggling with the inevitable decision over this period also was important. My mother's counselling gained from many years of experience working as a nurse, was immeasurable. Her words so carefully crafted made it possible for me to look at the situation objectively.

My siblings, Ben and Jennifer, were always around and provided encouraging support. We have always been a close family and this was invaluable in this time of crisis. I am aware that the decision also weighed heavily on my father. This was also a most difficult time for him.

There were other others who were my 'diamonds' at this time, such as my Auntie Christine in Adelaide and my cousin Bryn in Darwin, and of course, some of my dear friends.

While remaining terrified of the stoma and its aftermath, the light at the end of the tunnel was the fact that this operation was intended to allow my bowel to rest, and eventually it would be reattached and the whole digestive system would operate normally. This was the expectation and hope to cling to, and although it was not fully convincing at the time, it was all that was available. I was content to run with it.

Throughout this process, my primary surgeon was superb in assisting me in handling the crisis in my mind, and I was confident in the knowledge that if he felt there was another option rather than an ileostomy, he would have recommended it. But, given the failures of the past, there was also a reality to be acknowledged.

There was no guarantee of success even in this latest effort. To support and encourage me, he reiterated that this would be worth the effort, and should it work, it would be a wonderful bonus and give me the opportunity to live a normal life. Therefore, with or without any guarantees, this was a chance worth taking.

While agreeing to undertake the surgery, I never stopped searching for other options that may have been missed. Consequently, in the weeks leading up to the procedure, I investigated some probable medical alternatives that could avoid having to undergo surgery. One area was physiotherapy to strengthen my stomach muscles. The rationale was that if the muscles around the bowel area were made sufficiently relaxed, this would in turn relieve pain and perhaps moderate or even cease the incontinence.

Hence, I attended a number of sessions at a practice in South Brisbane, and was treated by a very skilful and caring physiotherapist. She gave me much encouragement as she attempted to resolve my lower abdomen issues and make me feel a lot better. Overall, the treatment, especially in the earlier stages, was most encouraging, as I always returned from the physiotherapy sessions feeling a little bit better each time.

As always, these feelings of relief were only temporary. There was no lasting impact on pain, incontinency or frequent visits to the toilet. This was again another disappointment.

At this point I accepted that perhaps the condition was irreversible, and I was destined to have the procedure for an ostomy as the only viable possibility. This was realistically the end of the line.

Emerging at this time, mostly around the fears surrounding the ileostomy, was also a problem with my mental state. My GP thus referred me to Lily Studios based at Indooroopilly in Brisbane. This practice comprises a group of psychologists who provide counselling services around the many personal and emotional hurdles that women face in their daily lives. Interestingly, Lily Studios also assisted women with anxiety issues because of physical changes to their bodies. This was consistent with my reactions at the time given that I was overcome with the growing anxieties over the impacts of the impending surgery on my physical appearance. In my emotional state I misconceived this as disfigurement.

With Lily Studios I could discuss my fears and obtain feedback on my emotions. This became important, as then I was able to understand the complex personal nature of my emotions and fears, and to develop different strategies to confront the problem. Acknowledging that the challenges I faced from a personal perspective were huge, and not every issue was effectively addressed, I am grateful for that counselling. It provided a small step forward in coping with many of the anxieties that were so overwhelming. I recommend this type of therapy for someone faced with a surgical intervention that can be intimidating.

With the surgery fast approaching, the idea of living with a stoma, and the challenges to the practical side of daily life, were still very much an unknown quantity. While I had some general knowledge about stomas drawn from the Web and the many books and pamphlets that were freely available, there was still much to learn.

Closer to the surgery and taking the advice of my GP, I attended a local clinic at the Holy Spirit Hospital in Spring Hill, Brisbane, to understand and practise the daily processes of maintaining the stoma. This included cleaning and changing the bag, and specific instructions on managing the integrity of the unit to prevent leakages. A major component of the tutorial classes and onsite demonstrations was obviously the hygiene, as the effects of infection caused by poor practices could lead to other health issues. Attention to this detail is probably most important in preventing infection, especially when considering the many activities that ostomates can be regularly involved in.

At the day clinic at the Holy Spirit Hospital, I met Pat, a stoma nurse who was very experienced in working with patients on stoma management. Pat is an excellent stoma therapy nurse and a very comforting person who offered support, guidance and confidence in managing a stoma before and after surgery. While many of my personal anxieties were still around, meeting her became very important in developing an increasing level of confidence in tackling the confronting realities that lay ahead. I cannot thank people such as Pat enough for all the assistance provided during my visits to the Holy Spirit Hospital.

It was now time to face my fears head on.

Chapter 6

The Life-Changing Surgery

Expose yourself to your deepest fear; after that,
fear has no power, and the fear of freedom shrinks
and vanishes, you are free.
– Jim Morrison

It was October 2011. Having worked at Virgin Airlines for about ten years and endured so many difficulties, the time of reckoning had arrived. As a final gesture, and as a reassurance as well as justification for the decision to proceed, I reminded myself that to date everything possible had been attempted and now there was nothing to lose. It was time to get on with it.

My future prospects in the airlines were also influential in the decision to proceed with the surgery. While the concerns about having a stoma and the influence this would have on my relationships with workmates still endured, the position at Virgin was always the job of my choice. The surgical option did provide me with some hope that if successful, and an adequate fix to most of the problems could be found, I could resume this cherished career.

Just prior to the operation my morale received an unexpected boost. I was attended by an admitting nurse called Karen who talked to me about the impending surgery, and other matters relating to the procedure. I asked the usual questions patients ask, but I suspect that mine were laced with high anxiety, fear and dread. Perhaps Karen actually felt the pain and mental anguish. She spontaneously lifted part of her clothing and exposed an ileostomy bag. That totally caught me off guard – it was truly a defining moment.

Karen was a registered nurse who was a few years older than me and through different circumstances was also afflicted with a bowel disorder. Karen had been a para-legal working in a law firm in Brisbane when she was diagnosed with Crohn's Disease. Crohn's is a chronic inflammatory bowel disease that is characterised by redness, swelling and pain within the digestive track. In many instances, inflammation can develop anywhere along the gastrointestinal track, even starting from the mouth of the sufferer and extending to the anus. In effect, it is a very debilitating condition for the sufferer. Karen's condition was one where she had to endure multiple corrective surgeries, not dissimilar to my experience, with few positive outcomes to show for all the efforts. Like myself, following these multiple surgeries, Karen also ended up with an ileostomy.

Unbelievably, I was engaging with a person who knew about my anguish. Most importantly, she was someone I could trust because she shared so much common ground through her own personal experiences.

Indeed, meeting Karen was serendipitous, as she could comfort me at the crucial time before this frightening and life-changing surgery. In a lightbulb moment, she instilled in me the fact that when emboldened with pure resilience and a commitment to take it on, the ileostomy can be turned around to become a process of discovery for the individual. Once this occurs, normality could be achieved by anyone who gives it their best shot.

During our discussions, Karen mentioned the care and compassion given to her by others within the medical profession. Her belief was that without this help her life would otherwise been much more difficult. That experience engendered a desire to help others in medical distress and was the catalyst driving her towards a nursing career.

After surgery and during the course of recovery, I was also nursed by Karen and seeing her around during this period as my strength returned, kindled my will to fight on.

My surgery took place at The Wesley Hospital and was performed by my primary surgeon. I remember even at the moment prior being taken to theatre still feeling very apprehensive and somewhat terrified. My mind was constantly working overtime, debating back and forth why a thirty-one-year-old like myself should be having an appendage attached to her body. While locked in this mode, thoughts began revolving on the next set of emotions that would surface when awaking after the procedure, and looking down at myself and *seeing this awful thing*.

Most importantly at this time were the surgeon's encouraging words on the opportunities to be gained relating to quality-of-life issues. These had a calming effect, and gave me much-needed positive reinforcement. They became the catalyst in bringing together the thoughts resonating about improving my life and even the prospect of motherhood, and then rationalising that all of this would not be possible without the surgery. In every sense they brought together my yearning for a longer and much better existence. Hopefully this procedure would fulfill all the desires that I had been craving since the age of eighteen.

After fifteen years of pain and despair, a possible ultimate solution to solving my problem was now at hand.

The operation was performed laparoscopically and my first reaction on awakening, and while still somewhat groggy, was to confirm the expected result of the operation. I lifted the bed sheet and looked down the length of my body towards the waist, and there it was, the so-dreaded bag, together with all the tubes and the connections to other parts of the body. While this was anticipated following the pre-operation counselling and the advice received, it was still a moment of despair. Adding to the already existing high anxiety levels of overflowing emotions, and feeling absolutely devastated, that was now a different me. I burst into tears. It was indeed very difficult to discard the reality about not being a normal person. It was now a fact that I would not be able to go to the toilet as a normal person. At that very instant of seeing all the evidence of the surgery, the support, assistance, and words of encouragement provided by so many kind people prior to the surgery, had little or no effect.

Throughout all of this I retained a glimmer of hope that the surgery was a work-in-progress and with the resting of the bowel there was some reasonable chance of success. So, at this point, focus was directed towards the eventual removal of the stoma, the reattachment of the bowel, and of course normality.

This expectation was clearly something to cling to, but was

still tenuous, as in the recesses of my mind there was limited confidence in believing such a favourable outcome would occur. In contemplating the realities objectively, I began to accept that full recovery was perhaps a bridge too far, and that I was destined to be different. Mind numbing as this was, there was little choice but to be prepared for this different phase of life.

Once again, at this critical time Ben was a great comfort and support, even though it must have been very difficult and heartbreaking for him to witness my trauma. He took this all on, encouraging me all the time, dismissing as best he could his own emotional pain and personal turmoil.

In all of this, my parents were constantly at my side. Like my husband they also worked through their distress, as it was not easy to see this happen to one of their daughters. Looking back, it is difficult to envisage how I would have endured the anguish related to the introduction of the stoma without the support of my husband, parents, and of course the rest of the family together with some close friends.

I spent eight days in hospital recovering from the surgery, and while being cared for in recovery, I cannot speak more highly of the stoma therapy nurses in Ward 5E of The Wesley Hospital in Brisbane. They were precise and methodical as they reinforced the earlier lessons on managing a stoma, bag-handling and the importance of hygiene, not only at home but also in daily life.

As a new stoma patient, I learned that the proper functioning of the unit relies on the output into the bag, and in particular that the flow of waste is smooth and consistent. To ensure this occurred on a daily basis, I was advised on suitable diets, the choice of foods. I learned to avoid high-fibre diets because of their propensity to create blockages and limit or restrict the flow of waste. Most importantly, I had to avoid the incidence of bowel obstructions. Indeed, these obstructions can have serious and sometimes devastating effects. This is something I discovered some six years down the track when I nearly lost my life and unborn child due to this very condition.

Another important issue was leakage, which can be a very disconcerting. The very thought of a leakage can be frightening. Imagine the sight presented by the wetness of clothing in a social or work situation, and the embarrassment for the stoma patient as well as those in attendance. Adding to this is the fact that the discharge is waste and potentially very confronting to all, including the stoma patient.

Because leaks are an impost in the daily life of an ostomate, detailed attention and instructions are given by the stoma therapy nurses in the management of these unwanted events. The primary aim is focused not necessarily in stopping them, but managing them. Without any doubt, the best-case scenario would be the elimination of leaks; however, we await new ideas and innovations before this can happen.

When I say that being a stoma patient places one in a new world, I really mean it. Once a stoma is created, the patient is introduced to a plethora of different products to assist in everyday life. These include different types of bags, seals, thickening agents, adhesives and, importantly, deodorants. The challenge for new patients is to make themselves totally familiar with these products and their functions, and always to use them effectively.

I am not joking in saying that there is something for every stoma patient.

Having a stoma means that that one does not use the toilet like an ordinary person. In daily life these products are essential and a lifeline for stoma patients. They must always manage personal stocks of the products and replenish them well ahead of time. I always make it a priority to be in contact with the suppliers to ensure that the products are available, especially for any unforeseen emergencies.

In discussing product sourcing and availability, it is important to note that patients in Australia with stomas and other appendages are well served through our health system via easy access, usually at little or no cost. Once on a visit to Vancouver in Canada, due to an oversight and poor management on my part, I ran out of supplies and needed to access bags and other items. I was forced to replenish the products at considerable cost. I then learned that even for a Canadian citizen these products are only available at some cost. As a stoma patient, one has to be thankful for living in Australia, and very appreciative that our health system strongly supports ileostomy and colostomy patients.

So, now in post-surgery and armed with all the information, all the education and all the good advice given by so many compassionate and highly skilled professionals on living a normal life, I was discharged from The Wesley Hospital to continue the recovery process.

I was eager to return to my position at the airlines, but from medical advice it was clear that I needed more recovery time to deal with the challenges ahead, both physically and mentally.

From the physical aspect there was a need to adjust to the changes affecting my daily routine, which required gaining familiarity with the operations and nuances of my new waste management system. Engaging in this process centred on making the necessary adjustments and then to feel comfortable about them. The extra time away from work was certainly worthwhile.

Naturally in this process, I made some mistakes along the way, but these were generally considered as work-in-progress. Soon, I was well on the way towards adapting to the physical changes and feeling prepared to recommence my working and social life.

There were emotional and mental challenges, centred mostly around the realisation that in some ways I was not the same person anymore. Therefore, many of these emotions were still very much in play. Overall, in adapting to the changes, there was little choice but grudgingly accept the reality that I was now not a normal woman, and in wrestling with so many conflicting thoughts, stability became increasing difficult. Repeatedly, there was still the burning issue about my looks, how to dress and how to present myself in public. And as the fears and anxieties kept rising to the top, I had many feelings of depression resulting in tears. With this accumulation of issues, as well as others, there were many days during the recovery period where I felt almost overwhelmed.

At the back of my mind, I worried whether the procedure would be successful because of the poor results in the past. The possibilities of another failure were really problematic because this would entail a more different or drastic approach to address the problem. If it was unsuccessful then the large bowel would be removed and the stoma would become a permanent fixture. This issue became troubling throughout the recovery stage.

All of these matters were unnerving because other difficult decisions could likely be confronting me shortly. In many respects, it seemed that this phase was merely kicking the can further down the track, and another challenging and difficult decision with more profound impacts would have to be made. This was the situation in front of me as I began the life of an ostomate.

All that has since occurred was done with my consent, and it was now time to come to terms with all the outcomes of my decision. I needed to accept full responsibility and work through and accept all the eventualities unfolding. This was a difficult time, despite the positive sides to the surgery, because there were still more creeping doubts about having the ileostomy and a stoma, and of course the burning issue of the uncertain long-term prognosis. These were matters yet to be resolved as I stepped into a new world.

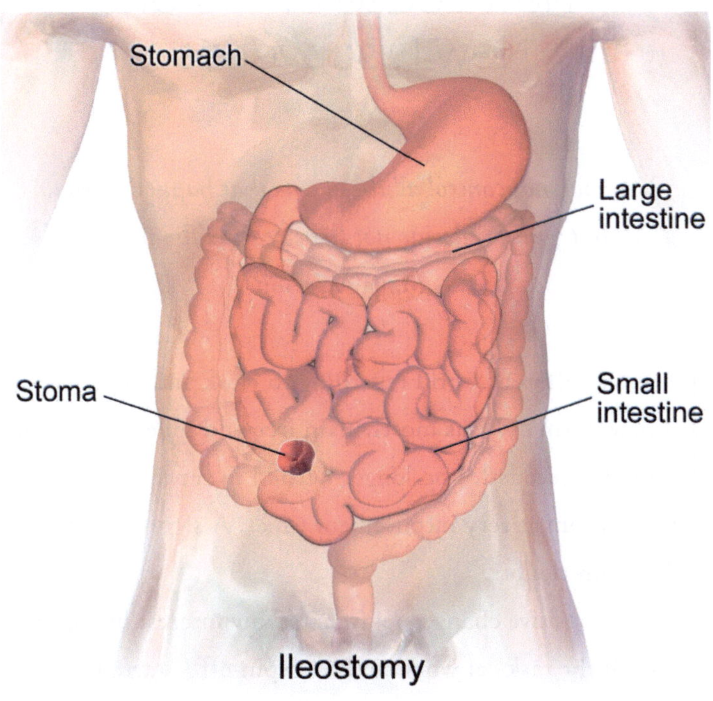

Figure 1: A stoma and ileostomy.

Chapter 7

A New Lease of Life and New Discoveries

You may not control all the events that happen to you, but you can decide not to be reduced by them.
— **Maya Angelou**

It was a different world returning to work and experiencing a new normal. I was mostly pain free and toilet frequencies had also receded. I no longer needed to repeatedly dash to the washroom at very inconvenient times. A significant change without any doubt.

These positive changes rejuvenated my interest in engaging across all the tasks at work, and as a spin-off I started to enjoy my days and slowly gained added job satisfaction. The feeling at this time was almost magical, and uplifting in that many of the shackles restricting my life had finally been shaken off. It was time to begin immersing myself more fully in the job, advance in the organisation, and achieve my objectives of a long career in the airline industry.

It is remarkable the positive changes that occur when a person is well rested and able to complete normal daily chores. Being pain free and without the need to use the toilet frequently, I was able to sleep well and hence feel much less weary confronting each work day. I also was far less impacted by the late finishes and early starts. Through gaining strength of mind and body, I became optimistic about achieving my goals.

To live a normal life, I had to manage the stoma. For example, I had to perfect the art of servicing the waste bag in a busy work environment. This took a little time and by adopting a trial-and-error process, I learned how to recognise the physical signs when the bag needed attention, and a trip to the restroom was warranted.

Being aware was quite easy, as emptying and servicing the bag was not dissimilar to the process involving any person using the toilet. This capacity to 'regulate' myself made me feel closer to being a normal person, albeit with some limitations. Overall, given the history of my illness, it is difficult to articulate what normal signifies except to say that there was great elation when I suddenly had the capacity to do many of the mundane activities at will that others generally took for granted.

Over the extended period, and in the attempt to engage in a busy lifestyle, there are essentially two major areas that require constant vigilance for a stoma patient. The first and most important is the impact of dehydration, a matter that must never be neglected. This is because without the assistance of the large bowel, the body does not absorb fluids readily, as occurs in a fully functioning digestive system. From an anatomical perspective, the small intestines or small bowel, are less efficient in performing this function. Therefore, without the large bowel it becomes critical that sufficient amounts of water are consumed by an ostomy patient to allow the small bowel the opportunity to absorb as much fluid as possible.

Generally, fluid consumption and how this can affect an ostomate, sometimes adversely, is a learning process. Speaking from experience, in the early days, there was an occasion when I became severely dehydrated leading to a trip to the emergency clinic at the hospital. Dehydration can have serious health consequences including life-threatening damage to the kidneys if not addressed quickly.

To explain this unwanted event in detail, it occurred following an upset stomach resulting in an excess discharge of fluids into the bag, and as this progressed, dehydration occurred in a severe way. In this instance, rather than address the matter immediately, I decided to continue unabated, which then made me very unwell after two days. As this condition deteriorated, I could not continue normal activities, and after delaying the inevitable, decided to seek proper medical assistance. In the emergency ward, while attached to intravenous fluids, the attending specialist told me it was indeed fortunate I was admitted at the time. He was quick to point out that delaying medical attention any further in the current situation could have resulted in some permanent damage to my kidneys. Besides the warnings of the doctor, my family and particularly my husband were exceptionally vocal about my lack of personal care and firmly admonished me about my slackness in managing the condition. The lesson here is to take no chances with dehydration, irrespective of the circumstances.

The second issue is being careful about the type of food

consumed. As my fellow ostomates will know some foods will initiate digestive problems and others not. I quickly learned which foods to consume and which to avoid. Adding to the need to be circumspect about the choice of food, it is also necessary to be careful in choosing foods that do not disrupt the functionality of the stoma and its output. In practical terms, foods that have fibrous strings are ones that should be avoided. Those fibres have the tendency to clog up the stoma hindering its ability to function properly, which is to empty the contents from the small bowel into the waste bag. Examples of foods with high fibre are certain green vegetables, and oranges. When a blocked stoma occurs, it is generally difficult for the patient to clear the blockage, and if the situation perseveres, then medical support is the next resort. Quite clearly a non-functioning stoma can be problematic and sometimes life threatening.

Fortunately, I have never experienced the device being totally blocked and requiring medical intervention. On a number of occasions, however, I suffered partial blockage. I then had to stand for a prolonged period under the shower allowing the free flow of water, as well as the natural action of the small bowel known as the peristaltic movement to clear the obstruction. This method worked in my favour and I have adopted this process as a useful course of action when necessary. Thank goodness for that.

In living with a stoma, whether temporary or permanent, different strategies are constantly being attempted to manage the stoma as best using trial-and-error. In looking for new ways I regularly check for research articles from magazines as well as the internet. Additionally, there is also a flow of personal blogs from my fellow ostomates which have been very helpful, and from these sources I have learnt a lot. As I am not afraid to try something new, I have applied many of the different ideas suggested in an effort to improve my quality of life. A big thank you to all who have expended so much of their time in spreading their message through the numerous information platforms available in the print and digital world.

Another support group is the medical people themselves, whom no doubt my fellow ostomates will wholeheartedly agree are a wonderful resource. I refer here in particular to the nurses and therapists, using their experience to assist and enhance the wellbeing of ostomates.

While I spent a lot of time developing and innovating best practices in living with an ileostomy to achieve a sense of normality, it was also a time to think about what lay ahead given the stoma was deemed to be only temporary. Superimposing all the positives of living with the ileostomy was the reality that the stoma may in fact become permanent. Should this happen, it would then totally change my life forever. In the short term I managed to deflect these concerns by pushing away all these thoughts. At the time, this was a rather small consolation. However, it was helpful in keeping a balanced mindset, and enough to enjoy the freedom afforded by the recent surgery. But I was still anxious about the long-term prognosis and, as I will outline in Chapter 9, the biggest challenge was yet to come.

As mentioned earlier, work became so much easier with less attention paid to managing the intricate balance between working and having to retreat in haste from the workstation. For the very first time in years, I was free from my impediments and able to take my place alongside my peers as a fully contributing Virgin employee, feeling destined for greater opportunities in this, the job of a lifetime.

On many occasions I was quite euphoric about my newfound freedom, which made me very upbeat and appreciative about all that was happening, unlike in the very recent past where survival was front and centre in my life. I was now at the point of enjoying my time at Virgin, relishing the startling change from being a sick person to a well person. This was a huge difference in a very short time and truly a very welcome feeling of total relief.

As my confidence grew, I began to feel mentally stronger, aided by the knowledge that the surgery was yielding so many positives, and with it came an increasing resilience in facing any perceived difficulties that may lay ahead. Indeed, this was a significant turnaround from the time all this began in 1996, when as a young adolescent I was thrown into an adult world, having to make decisions that were well beyond my comprehension.

There is little doubt the osteotomy was the main difference, and a significant factor that assisted and enhanced the fighting spirit that now emboldened me. Having the ileostomy and the improvement in the quality of my life, it was now possible to embrace the feeling of being a new person. I became more adventurous, accentuated by being more mobile and freewheeling. Overall, this quality-of-life issue cannot be overstated, because my life until this latest surgery was distinctly in two different descriptors, namely before and after ... perhaps also, terrible and wonderful.

One reason for writing this book is my hope that this experience will provide a positive framework for all those looking at, or agonising about, committing to an osteotomy or a similar surgical procedure. Here, my simple advice is that when evaluating your options always carefully consider the quality-of-life issue, as the 'after' solution described above is certainly a special outcome well worth looking forward to.

As the ileostomy created a new lease of life, my advice to fellow ostomates is to grab the opportunity with both hands as an important step in trying to live a normal life. A word of caution, because in saying this, it is worth remembering that amid all the positives, there are days of total frustration which invariably occur with incidents such as the occasional bag leak, skin irritations and, more seriously, a bout of gastro. Despite these setbacks, I have found that with the right approach, these inconveniences can be overcome especially when realising the main prize of normality and freedom are gifts much too valuable to ignore. And again, to reinforce the point, it is my belief that in keeping the right frame of mind, setbacks can become issues of relatively minor adversity, and not an impediment to the long-term goals of the ostomate.

With more confidence and newfound freedom, I began to look at opportunities for travel, and being an airline employee, use the perks available to facilitate flights. Soon after the surgery, Ben and I travelled extensively throughout Australia. These trips acted as a test run of the stoma, and its resilience across changing conditions. It was also an examination of my capacity to cope with the management of its intricacies under different travel conditions. In these endeavours, lessons were quickly learned in adapting to changing environments and situations, and along the way I coped easily with some mishaps and accidents. Fortunately, none of these caused any embarrassment. *But, so what if they did?* The priority of an ostomate is physical wellbeing above anything else.

By 2011, I had already worked at Virgin Airlines for more than ten years and was eligible for long service leave. Having road-tested myself with those trips around Australia, and feeling confident about my ability to travel with a stoma, Ben and I were on our way to Canada.

My trip to Canada was to Vancouver via Los Angeles, a journey of about around nineteen hours. Being my first attempt overseas, I was full of trepidation as there were stoma bags to empty, particularly in the first sector of the trip, which was more than thirteen hours. Even though I had some confidence built by the earlier flights, there were still the inevitable *what if* questions such as what if the bag broke open in mid-flight. I would have to access a toilet quickly and the issue would become problematic especially if this urgency clashed with peak demand for these facilities.

Another related issue was the fact that it was necessary to be watchful about when to use the toilet, given the length of time needed to ensure the necessary procedures for the detachment and attachment of the device. I must admit, even to this day, the issue relating to the emergency use of the toilet in a peak-demand scenario has never been resolved because it has never happened. However, I am more confident in dealing with this matter if it occurred.

From experience, I now know that these issues were really anxieties of a different mindset, leading to a level of fear rather than a reflection of reality. In fact, I would suggest that for ostomates travelling on planes, the chances of experiencing these *what if* problems would be very rare. Therefore, from my perspective, I have full confidence in the integrity of the equipment on any trip taken, whether within Australia or abroad. My last word to ostomates on this subject is: *Do not be fearful, as with proper care you will always get through. Enjoy your travel at all times!*

My trip to Canada was most memorable. I spent some time with my aunt Amanda in Vancouver and travelled to many places. Another reason, and an important one for travelling to Canada, was to attend an education workshop in Toronto centred on a range of issues related to ostomies. This forum, *Living with an Ostomy*, was of particular interest, being my first exposure to such an event outside Australia. The workshop was also an opportunity to be introduced to new ideas and information that would assist in my life as an ostomate.

Another compelling reason for attending was the presence of Jessica Grossman, a Canadian who was, and is still, very prominent in various media platforms, and she acts as an advocate for ostomates. Jessica, a digital marketer with an ileostomy herself, is internationally well known for her website *Uncover Ostomy*.

This forum was set up to break down the stigma surrounding an ostomy, to spread positive awareness of the importance of this life-saving surgery, and to encourage body positivity for all those living with this condition. A point that Jessica makes is that hiding a stoma achieves no real purpose as it (the stoma) is still going to be there.

The workshops addressed real-life situations, best practices and perceivable outcomes for ostomates. It was a real eye-opener on many fronts. Discussion highlighted key elements and challenges, such as coping with grief and loss, anxiety, therapeutic relationships, body image, self-esteem, sexual intimacy, and strategies to address fear and rejection. Being a first-timer, my foray into the stoma world was a fantastic learning experience, with the knowledge gained becoming progressively important as I grew more familiar with my condition.

Looking back, my exposure to the educational workshop in Toronto was a vital phase in the adjustment process, and I thoroughly endorse the value of these medical support forums for stoma patients. At the time of writing this book there was a growing number of them occurring in many locations, particularly in the larger centres in Australia. I wholeheartedly advise attending these gatherings, which will provide a valuable education resource not only for ostomates, but for others involved in this area.

These workshops also benefitted me significantly because of the similarities to the stoma workshops at The Prince Charles Hospital in Brisbane. Working now as a registered nurse, and as an ostomate, I am a regular presenter at these workshops. I still regard my Toronto experience as a valuable contribution to my ongoing journey, where I seek to reinforce the message of resilience and to engender long-term advocacy on behalf of ostomates.

Meeting Jessica Grossman was a special moment for me. My

first impression was her positiveness even though she herself had a debilitating bowel condition. During the forum we met on more than one occasion, and during each conversation I found her attitude so infectious that it was almost impossible not to become galvanised towards thinking and visualising the future possibilities and outcomes that I could attain.

My discussions with Jessica were a catalyst in turning around my built-in perceptions and fears about living with a stoma bag. To explain this more fully, at this time I was still very conscious of the bag and felt strongly this was a major handicap and stigma. My reactions, due mainly to embarrassment and fear of rejection, led to the tendency to avoid any discussion on the subject. This is common among people with these devices. Meeting Jessica immediately changed this attitude. She explained that while an ostomy was a reality, there were many positive ways to live, citing powerful examples that had yielded conclusive and discernible improvements in the public life of an ostomate. She was convincing in her view that there was no reason for an ostomate not to be open and comfortable, and be able to discuss the issue without fear or embarrassment.

In her view, the key in engaging in openness is adopting a sense of positivity about the medical condition, always emphasising the point that if you come out and tell people about it and say *this is what I have and I'm fine with it,* then people see it positively.

Conversely, she says that if you go up to someone and say *there's this gross weird thing attached to me,* everyone else is going to see the same thing. Then people will automatically come to see it as some sort of disability.

Jessica was diagnosed with Crohn's Disease while very young and between the ages of eleven and thirteen she was bedridden in hospital. She was unable to eat due to the pain, and unable to move due to weakness in her body. Also, she bled excessively from her bowels. *Imagine your insides having sharp knives grinding through them constantly. That was my life.*[1]

After countless diets, multiple tests and medications with their side effects, Jessica had to make a life-saving choice. The doctors told her that unless she had the surgery, her life would be in jeopardy. In 2003, at the age of thirteen, Jessica underwent an ileostomy as her last hope. With this surgery there was a turn in her fortunes. Jessica has generally been in good health ever since, and she was able to carry on with her life by completing high school, obtaining an undergraduate degree at the University of Western Ontario and a Masters at New York University. She has also gained professional recognition and business status by setting up and running her own digital marketing agency in Toronto, which has developed a unique online community. It is a web interface allowing ostomates around the world to come together and exchange ideas, share tips and discuss issues.

I frequently use this website, as well as others, as a resource to update my information on the important issues and events. I recommend the initiatives of Jessica Grossman through her website uncoverostomy.org as a significant resource for those living as an ostomate.

Ostomates can face many different hurdles in their lives, particularly in the case of the long-term prognosis being poor.

1 *Western Gazette*, Volume 104, Issue 98, 7 April, 2011.

Therefore, taking one step at a time should be viewed as a positive move, and a crucial stage in gaining confidence for the long road ahead. In my case, attending the workshop in Canada and meeting Jessica were the small steps I took moving forward. As Jessica had faced similar decisions as myself about the long-term prognosis, I believe my interactions with her and all the positive vibes received were of major assistance when I approached the more difficult decision to undergo further surgery.

One of my biggest gains from the interactions was strengthening my belief I could do anything with my life irrespective of the ostomy. This was a journey of self-discovery that having an ostomy was not the end of the world, and it gave me the freedom to do things, never thought possible before, such as climbing Mount Edith Cavell in the Canadian Rockies, and visiting many parts of the United States and Europe.

This is not to say I was thrilled about the idea of living with an ileostomy, but to a large extent this has been countered by working hard at focusing on the things that have been gained and not what has been lost.

Similar to others who have undergone ostomy surgery, there are the good days of being really grateful for having the surgery, and days of total frustration and the desire to be as far away from stomas as possible. As my fellow ostomates may agree, these are the days when the bag leaks, the skin becomes irritated, and days where it is a struggle to keep oneself hydrated to avoid the usual bad headaches, dizziness, and severe body cramps. Added to this, a bad outcome is being admitted to hospital emergency with several bags of intravenous fluids attached to your arms.

Then there are also the days where one is truly unlucky by being inflicted with gastro and its aftermath.

While contending with the annoyances described here, it was still important for me to continue to look for innovations, or new information that would assist individuals in their daily lives. Every three years, the International Ostomy Association organises World Ostomy Day on the first Saturday of October. These worthwhile events provide updated information to enhance the life of ostomates. As well, online information through Google and other sources are readily available.

In seeing myself as one of a number of advocates aiming to promote ideas and programs, I am always seeking further initiatives that will increase community awareness about ostomates. For example, on a visit to Japan in July 2016, I stumbled across a designated ostomy toilet at Tokyo's Narita Airport. Although at the time it seemed a novelty, it is a step in the right direction, and encouragingly another level of recognition within the broader society. So, there is hope that at some point this idea will be replicated in Australia.

As I continued in this phase of a new lease of life and on the path of discoveries, my attention turned back to work. This was stimulated by my wanting to get more out of life. After all the years of difficulty and disappointment, I believed the time had arrived for me to accomplish something worthwhile.

With the freedom given me by the ileostomy, I had the opportunity to achieve higher goals, and this was now attainable at the airline, with my proficiency also increasing markedly. I continued to plough on with little in mind except to work in my dream job, not knowing that before long there would be a distinct change in priorities and attitude towards the workplace, and events that would channel my life in a completely different direction.

Chapter 8

Rebooting my Career

All the darkness of the world cannot extinguish the light of a single candle.
— St Francis of Assisi

Returning from overseas and now heading towards my thirteenth year at Virgin, I wanted to reclaim all that was lost because of the years of illness. With my newfound freedom, while much of my attention was still focused towards the possibilities of my long-term advancement with the airlines, there was also this feeling that in reality working in the industry was somewhat different from my earlier perceptions and expectations. Yes, the industry had given me some great moments, but somewhere deep in the recesses of my mind was this changing belief that the career path now lacked enough abundance in the sense of being truly fulfilling. There must be more to life and work than travel and tourism.

This matter of abundance was influenced by the people I encountered, and in many instances who cared for me during the very difficult times. Looking at the way those people went about their work, their dedication, commitment, and strength of conviction, I began to have thoughts of new directions and opportunities.

So, despite being comfortable in my work, there were a number of compelling reasons for fostering a change in my attitude.

An important factor was the time lost as a result of being absent through surgery and general illness. Because of those lost years I was well behind many of my peers, so that promotion would be harder despite the improvement in my health, and my newfound capacity to become more immersed in the job.

I was still confident in my work performance. Indeed, it was good, especially in respect to my technology skills, which were very sound in resolving myriad issues relating to travel. I was considered very useful in the day-to-day demands of the workplace, especially in the use of my conflict-resolution skills. However, it was clear that I was going nowhere while I saw my peers move upwards in different trajectories. Never one to deny the success of others, I was always pleased for them; however, witnessing my lost opportunities with limited chances to make up lost ground was still very difficult.

I felt left behind as a forgotten person and marking time in the organisation. If this was the case then there was little or no purpose in remaining.

Adding to this dilemma, there was still the overriding question of the long-term prognosis associated with the recent surgical procedure. The still unanswered question remained about the end game. The preferred outcome was the full repair and restoration of the bowel, but this was not at all guaranteed.

At that time, it was nothing more than wait and see in the

hope that a full recovery, and the chance of a normal life was just around the corner. The reality, however, was much different, as the medical intervention was undertaken on the basis of a trial, and with so many unknowns came deep uncertainty as to whether my life would continue its temporary upward trend.

In this new phase, I was now facing a waiting period, being fully aware that should this current corrective action not resolve itself, then other more confronting and difficult decisions would need to be made. Knowing full well all the possible outcomes, good and bad, that could result from the procedure, failure and its consequences remained an unthinkable proposition. On these grounds, and accepting the likelihood of encountering later difficulties leading back to the destructive lifestyle of the past twelve years, I questioned the value of continuing to work in the travel industry. Any thoughts of repeating the recent past were totally unacceptable and became the final catalyst in considering alternative employment possibilities, whether the worst- case scenario of surgical failure was to occur or otherwise.

Another consideration, but one of lesser impact, was the cultural and business changes that were occurring in the airline, largely brought about by corporatisation and other economic influences. It became obvious from my perspective that the impact of these changes had now made working for the airline more impersonal, highly businesslike and less attractive.

Significantly and unexpectedly, my long dream of becoming an airline stewardess and the attraction of flying was suddenly no more. This change of attitude was largely brought on by battles with my health, but over time was also influenced by many conversations with my friends who were then working as hosties. It became apparent that the actual realities of their working lives and the personal pressures experienced by cabin crew while crisscrossing the continent and engaging in many hours of gruelling schedules were far from glamorous. It also became evident that the working conditions placed undue demands on their personal wellbeing, with the resultant spin-offs also impacting their immediate families. It is therefore not surprising that many of these friends working as cabin crew have since left Virgin Airlines.

It was time to recall the earlier words of wisdom given by my teachers at Mt St Michael's all those years ago: it is unwise to take too literally the idea of the rosy pictures of glamour and excitement that is widely perceived as the standard in the travel industry. The reality is starkly different in the sense that this apparent glamour occurs mostly at the top layers of management structures, and in actuality, what lies beneath is very different.

Hindsight is such a wonderful thing, but the teachers were right on the money with their assessment of the industry. My evolution in thought is clearly an example of how an individual's mindset and attitude can change from exposure to different experiences. When I left high school, I never envisaged that I would consider a career beyond the travel industry. The fact that I now sought change is a testimony to the idea that life itself, and its hardships, are sometimes great levellers in bringing forth a true appreciation of the new opportunities that are out there for the individual to explore.

As questions began to weigh on my mind about the long-term future, it was time to look at other options.

As I had a Diploma in Hospitality Management, coupled with my experience at Virgin Airlines, I looked for alternative employment in the hospitality industry such as in tour management, travel bureaus, hotels and in tourism retail outlets. These were all certainly viable options.

While exploring them, my mind kept circling back to another area of particular interest: health care. As a patient, my interactions with health care professionals through my illness were so significant that they had a major and lasting effect on me. In particular, the nurses and doctors were always warmly supportive and skilful in helping to resolve or mitigate my difficult health problems. There is certainly a truism in the words that people are great ambassadors for their professions, especially when their contributions have lasting and positive impacts. In particular, these lasting impacts come from people's individual abilities to perform well, not only in the area of technical skills and expertise, but importantly in their client-patient relationships. It was therefore in this context, and the cumulation of time spent in the care of health workers, that made me look closely at a career in this area.

I thought of my interaction with Karen before and after the stoma surgery. Our relationship was significant when I was struggling to come to terms with the challenges to my life and the future. I was fortunate to draw on her personal courage and strength, which were needed for the days and weeks when I was adjusting to the changes happening to my body. Starting with

Karen, other nurses and medical staff, I saw the immense value of their work.

Therefore, even from those very early days while in health care, there was the genesis of an idea that I would *love to do this,* and to do it in the best way possible. So, as it became clear that a change in career was in the wind, the opportunity to engage in a profession that assisted people with ostomies, and contribute to their wellbeing was foremost in my thinking. I firmly believe that if you can make a difference to just one person, then you have served the main purpose of your profession.

Why nursing?

Well, it is clear that when a person like myself spends so much time surrounded by hospital walls, a true appreciation of the nursing role and the integral part nurses play in obtaining a positive outcome for their patients is gained. In the hospitals while being cared for, I came to realise that they deserve much praise, because as a collective these nurses helped me greatly by their compassion and care. Seeing the dedication constantly displayed for their patients, sometimes under extreme circumstances and conditions, made a career in nursing very attractive to me.

Another influence in this choice was my mother, Ingrid. She has now retired, but had worked as a nurse for fifty years. Her experience was diverse and wide-ranging, having worked in hospitals in Adelaide, Melbourne and Brisbane. When I was a child and teenager growing up in Melbourne and Brisbane, her dedication and compassion were always on display for those who were entrusted to her care. Needless to say, in my time of crisis from the early days in 1996, Mum was always there to support, console and most of all, offer comfort while I struggled with pain and uncertainties for the future. It is obvious that her many years of nursing brought out the best in terms of her skills, and always to my benefit. Today Mum still remains my rock as I continue going forward with my life and career in nursing.

It would be remiss of me to not mention that the choice of nursing as a career was also influenced by my younger sister Jennifer. When I was considering leaving the airlines, Jennifer, or JJ as she is affectionally known, had already commenced a career as a midwife and was undertaking a degree in midwifery at the Australian Catholic University. Jennifer started out as a beauty consultant, and after realising that this sector had limited opportunities, decided that a change was required and embarked on midwifery. This was a real challenge for her, particularly as the course was uncharted territory, being so different and intense from beauty therapy. This was also a particularly tough decision for Jennifer, but she is now a successful midwife working at the Royal Women's Hospital in Brisbane.

As well, when mentioning that the medical profession runs in the family, I should add that my brother Ben is a qualified sonographer, and very much like his two siblings, has chosen this discipline after successful stints in other sectors.

So, by this time it was obvious that nursing would be the preferred choice. As a spin-off and of obvious interest, this move would give me not only the opportunity to assist people with stomas, but the possibility even at this stage of extending these skills and act as an advocate for ostomates. With the decision made, I started to review all the nursing courses available in the

Brisbane area and I selected the course offered at the Southbank TAFE, as an alternative to the one offered at the Queensland University of Technology.

With everything in place and emboldened with having established a viable option in terms of a new career, the time had now come to leave Virgin Airlines.

Do I miss the airline industry? The short answer is an emphatic *No*. Clearly with thirteen years already spent at Virgin, I had given it my best shot and accepted all its offerings, good and bad. I still view the time spent there as an achievement in the sense that it had provided the opportunity to satisfy an initial urge to work in my dream job. I was now in a position to say and feel that I have seen it all, or commonly referred to as been there, done that. It was clearly time to move on, to find a new beginning, to do something personally satisfying and challenging, and most of all to break new ground.

Having made the decision to leave, it must be said that the years spent at Virgin Airlines were invaluable in terms of the work experience and skills gained. I learned much about teamwork at the check-in desk, as it was the norm for individuals to coordinate and rely on each other, and develop the basis of good working and personal relationships.

In the airline sector attention to detail is a basic requirement for all tasks, because good practice always ensures that processes and procedures run smoothly and efficiently. This discipline was instilled in us from the very start, introducing a level of personal reliability and competency as invaluable assets that could be utilised whether in the airline industry or in other careers.

Customer relations and dealing directly with people on a one-to-one basis was a constant, and in this respect the airlines provided many valuable lessons about engaging with clients. A major lesson quickly learned was that while appropriate levels of empathy were always necessary, the practice of displaying firmness and fairness across the board were also essential to achieve a balance for all parties involved in transactions and disputes.

One point of difference, however, is that now working as a nurse, I am quite often faced with difficult situations that demand attention and remedial action. In these encounters, I sometimes reflect on my time at Virgin Australia where to satisfy a customer one would work through a computer checklist, and often tick and flick to resolve the problem. In my role as a nurse today it is difficult to do that as relationships and requests are much more personal, and enduring, therefore tick and flick always remains just a thought from an experience.

Chapter 9

Training with Intent

It seems to me that self-confidence and the ability to stand one's ground are essential if we want to succeed in life. I am not talking of stupid self-assurance but of an awareness of our inner potential, a certainty that we can always correct our behaviour, improve ourselves, enrich ourselves, and that things are never hopeless.

— Dalai Lama

Following in the footsteps of my mother and sister, and having explored all the options available, I undertook a nurses course at the Tertiary and Further Education campus, or TAFE. This was at the beginning of 2014 and I was able to begin the course without resigning from Virgin Airlines.

I chose not taking on the registered nurse course due to several reasons. Initially, I felt that enrolling immediately in a university course would be too difficult, incorrectly thinking at the time that attaining the academic standards would be difficult, given my only exposure to tertiary education was at the diploma level. This was a case of poor judgement, as my academic achievements in graduating from university after three years indicated otherwise.

It was evident I had sold myself well short when deciding on the pathway to train as a nurse.

Another important factor in play was that the TAFE course was much shorter, allowing a student to qualify within eighteen months. This timeframe was attractive because it reduced the financial burden on the family as I could return to the workforce on a full-time basis much sooner.

Being ill for so long was another reason for my choice. I was concerned that the stresses of university study could have an adverse effect on my health. While I had lived about a year with an ostomy, experiencing a new lease of life and mostly enjoying work with the airlines, there was still concern about underlying issues and uncertainty of my long-term prognosis. My main fear concerned unpredictable issues that would cause me to regress to the previous norm. If this were to occur it would take a heavy toll on my ability to successfully complete the three-year registered nurse course. Therefore, it seemed prudent to take a conservative approach and play it safe by enrolling in the shorter TAFE course. To underpin this decision, I also felt that in time there would be ample opportunity to upgrade the nursing certificate to a three-year course, and hence obtain a degree in nursing.

Another important issue was the ability to undertake part-time work to alleviate the financial burden while also studying. In this respect the TAFE course was attractive in that the smaller study workloads would allow for more part-time work compared to university study. Also influencing this decision was the opportunity to use my airline skills to secure work with an associate company of Virgin Airlines called Bluestone.

Bluestone was contracted to Virgin to supply check-in services for passengers travelling from Brisbane to domestic and international ports. Being experienced in all these areas, I was able to provide the required services. Seemingly this was going to be a win-win situation with the potential to work for Bluestone on an ongoing basis while studying. Unfortunately, this employment did not last past 2014, as the company ceased operations, and my financial position did not improve in any significant way.

Coming back to the TAFE course, I began study at the Southbank campus in Brisbane in February 2012. I remember fronting up on the first day, attending the classes and viewing the teaching modules that were on offer as part of the training program. My first impressions were that the facilities for training were excellent, and as the curriculum was generally a hands-on approach, the set-up included a full ward with all the modern equipment and gadgets one would expect to see in any working hospital. There was a lot to commend the training program, as the classrooms were well resourced and the teaching staff of high quality and experienced.

Filled with enthusiasm, I attended lectures and practical sessions, and in the initial stages I became somewhat comfortable moving in a completely different direction. However, in the weeks while slowly becoming immersed in the curriculum, and free to explore all aspects of the course, a few doubts began to creep in as to whether this program was actually the appropriate pathway to become a nurse and achieve my goals.

In evaluating the decision to start this course, my observations indicated clearly that the scope of practice for enrolled nurses was quite different from that of a registered nurse. I soon concluded that this was not an appropriate direction as it was not exhaustive enough in its content for one to engage in the broader range of areas when delivering health and patient care. It was certainly unlike the role my mother played in all her years working as a nurse.

Being unsure of the next move, I reviewed my decision and identified once again my motivations for a career change. This again triggered memories of the level of care afforded me throughout my illness, and the outstanding assistance given by nurses at hospitals during and after the many surgeries. As well, there were also the memories of unforgettable interactions with some nurses who inspired me to think that there was also a place for me in the medical world to contribute to others who were battling difficulties like mine. Gradually, the idea of being an advocate for ostomates began to take shape, and the view that acquiring these skills would be the way to transition and to specialise in this area. Although this was still some distance away, the possibility of teaching the subject was also an attractive proposition.

It became obvious that this TAFE course would not meet my goals. The capacity to work across a wider range of patient care required a more in-depth knowledge and proficiency around clinical and patient management skills, as well as a better understanding of pharmacology, physiology, anatomy and associated areas. My only recourse was to undertake the full registered nursing course offered at a university.

Having made the decision, I had to enrol in the university as soon as possible so as to move quickly and complete the qualifications within a reasonable timeframe. Waiting out the full year was not palatable, as such a move would mean that obtaining a qualification in nursing would take four rather than the mandatory three years. Unfortunately, with such poor timing it was well into May when I decided to make this change, and as a result it was too late to enrol at any university for the current semester. The only option was to apply for a mid-year enrolment. I chose the Queensland University of Technology (QUT), and commenced study in July of that year.

It immediately became evident that this move was the right strategy.

This course provided the opportunity to learn the appropriate skills and knowledge to achieve my goals. I felt really satisfied in knowing that my objectives in making this change were justified. Now there was the opportunity to develop my skillsets to assist patients undergoing problems similar to my own. Therefore, from the beginning of the course, I embarked on developing some specific strategies to achieve these goals.

Firstly, I felt that to be effective as an advocate for those suffering from various forms of bowel disease and similar disorders, it was important to understand more about its complexities, and hence be better informed of the medical and technical issues. In this context, it was going to be necessary to improve my knowledge in anatomy by drawing from more in-depth research into the curriculum presented in the course. Given my already existing interest in anatomy, and by exploring the subject further, I discovered more useful and practical information, and data outside the course guidelines.

To add to the mix was the need to build a competent approach to physical patient care, and in this respect learn as much as possible from practical demonstrations, which were plentiful throughout the course. Consequently, I learned much about the many aspects of bowel disorders, including problems associated with Crohn's Disease and cancer. This was invaluable when I was assigned to the surgical ward of the hospital to provide post-operative care to patients who had undergone bowel surgery leading to an ostomy.

At the personal level, I discovered that with more knowledge comes confidence. Consequently, I gained much satisfaction when engaging face-to-face with patients, especially to feel their warmth and gratitude after I assisted them. A wonderful experience all round.

To many of the patients, the idea of a bag as a waste disposal unit remained foremost in their minds even though most had already received some form of counselling prior to their procedure. In spite of that, the outcome still remained a traumatic event, and one that required appropriate skills on the part of a nurse when interacting with these patients. Because of my similar lived experience, I developed many good relationships with ostomates while I was still training.

By the final stage of the course, I was feeling very pleased that the decision to have the surgery had indeed yielded many positive outcomes. But during this short passage of time, I had to make some hard decisions, as the issue of the long-term prospects of the ileostomy and its ongoing health implications were to be addressed.

As mentioned previously, the initial idea of having an ileostomy was to give the bowel a rest for a short period, and then to re-attach it to the small intestine with the intention that the resting period would repair the problem. This would give the system the chance to function normally. I must admit, however, that instinctively I felt that a permanent ileostomy would be the most likely outcome. In other words, if re-attachment was not undertaken, the stoma would remain with me for the rest of my life.

Now having to confront another hard decision, there were further consultations with the surgeon on the options. While being told certain realities, and these truths are always difficult, no matter the circumstances, I was somewhat unprepared for the response. In his opinion, reconnection and removal of the stoma was not viable. He believed that the problems of the past would re-occur, leading to a cycle of surgeries of attaching and detaching the bowel, the latter being referred to as an anastomosis. In conversation, he referred to the existing mechanical defects of the bowel, and the possibility that being dormant, the chances of contracting cancer in the future was a matter to be carefully considered.

He thus recommended I should continue life with a permanent ileostomy with the removal of the large bowel after key-hole surgery. Initially he intended to perform a proctocolectomy, which was the removal of every part of the large bowel including the rectum. However, this was considered unsafe because the mesh from a previous surgery had now become embedded in the area, and surgery in this region could result in excessive bleeding and be life threatening. So, the safe option in this case was the removal of the bowel and keeping the rectum intact but stitched up. While feeling disappointed with the surgeon's recommendation, I found this advice easier to accept because generally life was better and more enjoyable. Important in this decision was that there was now little or no possibility of regressing to the life and traumas of the recent past. Having an ileostomy meant I was now free of pain, as there were no more brutal nights, there were no more frequent dashes to the toilet, and most of all I felt that my life was somewhat normal. I felt good and I enjoyed work and travelling.

The surgery was performed in 2014, and because there were no complications, recovery was much easier compared to previous procedures. It was now time to adjust, and it was only a short period after surgery that I began to feel more comfortable again. I was ready to move forward.

My nursing course also included an opportunity to undertake an overseas study assignment: a two-week trip to Indonesia to learn about its health care systems. There were ten places available across the health faculties, incorporating social science, physiotherapy, and three places allocated for nursing students. As places for those in nursing were limited, selection was on based on merit.

For me, this was an absolute bonus, with the exciting prospect of working in a foreign clinical setting, and obtaining some first-hand experience about a different health care system in a contrasting cultural setting. One of the key objectives of the study tour was to allow health professionals to gain more knowledge about these systems from an Asian perspective. As a flow-on effect, it was hoped that the program would build and contribute to an ongoing collaborative and inter-professional relationships between professionals of the two countries.

It was evident that the study program was going to be a challenging one. Indonesia was a developing country, and in interacting with its health care system, there would be exposure to some situations that would be very confronting, especially given the existing cultural and economic differences that exist. More interestingly, I felt that in looking at a career in health care, the visit to Indonesia would indeed be a chance to observe its health environment knowing that the overall quality of this care in Indonesia is well below that of Australia, and one that was poorly resourced. This program appealed to me, particularly due to my quest for lifelong learning. The end of the nursing course was in sight, and seemingly there was no better way to finish than through observing real-life situations in a different environment. The idea of participating in such a program was indeed exciting.

Like all other interested students, my application was thrown into the ring. I documented every conceivable argument I could think of to support my selection. Overall, I felt quite confident of my chances as I had achieved a creditable level of academic excellence with a grade point average (GPA) of 6.6 so far in the course. Adding to this, it was felt that my application would be viewed favourably as I had received three successive commendations from the dean for academic excellence.

In addition to listing my academic achievements, my application stated that because I was an ostomate, and had an interest in wound care, this personal experience could be used to assist others living with the same condition. I suggested there was an opportunity to relate my personal experience and couple this with the effective techniques already employed while training in the wards.

Very important in the decision to travel and spend time in Indonesia was the opportunity to test my ileostomy and the performance of my waste bag system in trying conditions, which would be alien to those in Australia. There was already some fear over leaving the shores and safety of Australia for a developing nation, given the negative information I had received about health care and quality of service. Hence, I viewed this trip with some trepidation, underpinned by the need to be well prepared for the challenge if selected to participate in the program.

I was now moving to the end of the course with the prospect of a trip to Indonesia ahead of me, followed by some mandatory assignments to be completed. On reflection, my career change was appropriate. I had embraced and relished the opportunities associated in providing health care rather than working in the commercial service sector. Most satisfying in this context was the chance to assist people with medical ileostomies and colostomies. I could see that there was more for me to give by being able to venture down this pathway.

The next stage of my life was now ahead of me.

Chapter 10

Preparing to Engage in a Lifelong Learning Experience

Believe you can and you are halfway there.
— **Theodore Roosevelt**

After much nail-biting, I learned I had been selected for the program in Indonesia and would be part of the study group departing in late-December 2014. I was obviously ecstatic. So now fully energised and in anticipation of overseas travel, I made plans to organise the details of the trip.

Then I hit the skids! I was horrified. I had overlooked something altogether. In many ways this was understandable because at that time the focus was totally directed on winning the scholarship. My thoughts were centred around the logistics associated with travelling to Indonesia, completing the assignment and then returning home hopefully feeling pleased with the milestone achievement. In the excitement of being selected, matters relating to the ileostomy had been overlooked, particularly its implications in relation to the potential risks while visiting a developing country. The study program was in Semarang, the capital of Central Java. I had not investigated the quality of medical support available there if a problem with the stoma occurred.

I immediately hit the fear button. Having a stoma would generate a range of complications, making visiting Indonesia downright difficult, if not impossible. At this point, and with the health risks involved, my fears started to compound to the extent I even thought about declining the scholarship. My overriding factor was the impulse not to leave the shores of Australia and instead cower in a familiar and safe environment.

With this uncontrollable emergence of negative emotions acting as a drag, I had to urgently redress the situation or fall by the wayside. I needed help and advice, but most importantly I had to work through and filter my concerns in a calm and rational manner. I had to identify each of my concerns and then address them accordingly.

The support and advice from others were the next steps in regaining the appropriate balance to my mindset.

Firstly, in addressing these concerns about travelling, I reviewed my current lifestyle, beginning at the time of first receiving the stoma to the present day. Looking back on all these, including bag leaks, blockages, frequency and duration of discomfort, I then identified whether each of the incidents was either traumatising or downright inconvenient. I analysed the impact of each event and recalled the action I took to resolve each medical incident.

After doing this evaluation, the picture that emerged indicated that none of the incidents relating to the stoma and waste bag were life threatening, or even required major medical interventions. In fact, in almost every circumstance, corrective action was effectively undertaken, and any medical interventions were minimal and relatively easily addressed by a quick check with the local doctor. Thus, I concluded that these fears were an over-reaction by an overactive mind. In short, I was being unnecessarily concerned about a life-threatening situation when in fact this was very much of a low risk.

Now that I felt more confident in planning the approaching trip, the next phase was to address and examine ways of reducing the risk of a major medical intervention and possibly hospitalisation. Developing preventive techniques was critically important, as the chances of catching infection was quite high and something to be avoided at all cost.

To avoid potential infection, as I was assigned to a community where access to suitable medical support may be problematic, I needed to take special care, and indeed be quite strict in following daily hygiene procedures. I had to be very selective in the choice of food to ensure the proper functioning of the stoma was not compromised.

Having identified the courses of action required to protect myself, I set about reviewing other matters to be addressed. I had to ensure adequate health insurance cover was in place. This was particularly important in terms of gaining access and treatment at reputable hospitals if required. I needed a policy that covered medivac if transportation back to Australia was needed.

Repatriation was always a major consideration, and I discussed this matter with the course coordinator at the university, and together we developed a plan to ensure that these arrangements would be in place if necessary. I also made sure I had additional insurance for the days spent in Indonesia, outside of the official study program.

Feeling more confident that the contingencies were in place should medical assistance be required, I then ensured that there would be an adequate stock of medical supplies including stoma bags, cleaning fluids and supplementary medication for the trip. Based on past experience, the best idea was to have double the amount required. The ostomate would find that the excess supply would provide a good backstop and induce a sense of peace of mind.

Another important consideration was that if these items had to be sourced when overseas, and assuming access and availability, they would usually cost much more, as I experienced in Canada. Therefore, this trip was made with double the required amount of product. Talk about overkill, but I was not going to take any chances.

With the departure date set for December, everything moved rather quickly, with much time set aside to organise the medical supplies and to speak to my doctor for advice, as well others to gain a better insight and likelihood of any unexpected events occurring. In this planning phase attention to detail was foremost. I spared no effort to obtain as much information as possible.

The next focus was the enhanced procedures to be adopted each day to clean the stoma and change the bag. All 'my comrades' with stomas and similar devices would understand that *being anal* about hygiene and cleanliness is everything. This is the best protection from infections that could lead to other unwanted problems. No one in their right mind would want an infection involving their stoma under any circumstances.

The main cause of infections, particularly of the gastronomical kind when travelling to developing countries, is the quality of the drinking water. Consuming bottled water is strongly recommended. In turning to the stoma, this is technically an open wound, and therefore washing and cleaning using normal potable water in Indonesia, as one would in Australia, is a risk that could potentially expose the wound to infection. Therefore, it became evident that I would also have to use bottled water to clean the stoma and the area around it while in Indonesia. Another hurdle had now been addressed.

A factor that assisted me in feeling more secure was the fact that Ben decided that he would also travel to Indonesia, and remain there while I was involved in the study program. This was significant as it was in a sense insurance, if something went wrong. Most important of all was the level of comfort knowing that there was family around should a medical decision be required. With the university also aware of my medical status, and willing to act in my interests, it became very reassuring that there were now two parties on the ground looking after me.

We decided that Ben would travel with me directly to Semarang, leaving me to participate in the program. He would then travel to Jakarta and indulge in his passion for photography, traveling around the countryside, but always within striking distance of Semarang, should an untimely crisis occur. At the end of the program, I would travel to Jakarta, spending a few days exploring the city, followed by a few days in Bali before returning to Australia.

I was now in a very comfortable mindset and started to look forward to the trip. I recognised full well the challenges that lay ahead, but somewhat confident that should any unexpected medical difficulties arise, there were sufficient contingencies in place to address them.

Having attended to the medical issues, it was now time to plan for the program itself. As an introduction to the work involved in Semarang, here are some details, together with a brief insight of the study tour.

The team comprised nine persons made up of four nurses, two psychologists, and three social workers, all being final year students in their respective courses. There was also a senior staff member supervising the students.

In preparation for the visit, we were required to participate in an introductory Indonesian language course, which was of great interest to me, having had limited exposure to any foreign language. Included in the language module was also an overview on the cultural issues and local practices that we would encounter. To facilitate this short course, assistance was provided by two team members who were Indonesian by heritage, spoke the language fluently, and who would act as translators.

We were constantly reminded that many of the situations that we would encounter would be very different, and outside the norms and practices consistent with our training. We were encouraged to view our opinions or assessments on various aspects of the Indonesian health system, within the context of existing limitations, be that the skill of the health workers, availability of resources and finances, and other related factors.

As a group, we were cautioned that it was going to be a very challenging time because those involved in delivering health services in the Australian environment are accustomed to a system that is relatively well funded. We have modern medical facilities and good supporting services.

Throughout the discussions, we were always reminded about the poverty in Indonesia and that most of the patients attending hospitals and clinics in the communities around Semarang were poor. I took the opportunity to research Indonesian poverty before leaving. This was useful when observing the role of the health providers generally and the interrelationships between the local nurses and their patients.

The stage was set and we all knew that this venture would be very different for each of us personally, but would surely be an enlightening experience.

I gathered all my academic notes and other equipment, as well as organised the usual travel arrangements to ensure arrival in Semarang in time to join the team. I was ready and the date for departure could not come quickly enough.

Ben and I boarded a Virgin Airlines flight in December 2014 for the five-hour journey to Semarang, transiting through Denpasar in Bali. In flight, it was difficult to balance my feelings of excitement and apprehension, and it was somewhat of a relief when we arrived in Semarang where the whole study team was gathered. It was time also to connect with my fellow student Fabiola.

As this was an intensive educational study program jointly organised by the university and key health officials in Indonesia, many Indonesian health professionals were participants, not only as advisors, but generously offering their homes to accommodate us. I was billeted with Fabiola in the home of Dr Yus Wanti, a very prominent individual in the local medical fraternity. It was comforting being in close contact with a doctor should any emergency arise.

At the airport, Fabiola and I were met by our host Dr Yus Wanti and her two daughters, Sesaria and Annisa, and the first impression was their friendliness and welcoming nature. Dr Wanti was the medical director at the RSUD Tugurejo Hospital in Semarang, and it was a good feeling being around someone who is a professional dedicated to helping the sick and the poor. Adding to the relief was the knowledge that Dr Wanti's husband was also a doctor of some prominence in the area, and therefore all my bases were covered.

I guess it is normal when arriving in a new country to be curious as to what lies beyond the airport and the first glimpses of Semarang. To this end, Dr Wanti and her two daughters did not disappoint, driving Fabiola and me around on a Cook's tour of urban Semarang.

In this short tour, my first impressions of Semarang were rather like those experienced while travelling in Malaysia with my family. There were a lot of similarities between the two countries, except in my opinion that Malaysia seemed slightly ahead in its development, albeit with a significantly smaller population and land area.

We saw the old and the new Semarang on display. Naturally, as Indonesia is a Muslim country, the Grand Mosque was one of the first places we drove past. This is a wonderful piece of architecture, and looking at its grandeur and prominence, I started to understand the importance of the religion in the daily lives of its people.

On this outing we saw many other interesting sights, notably the Old Dutch neighbourhood, or Oude Stad, a reminder of colonial times when the Dutch ruled Indonesia. This area included many old buildings that were slowly being restored. This visit was interesting in the light of my Dutch heritage, and the knowledge that my maternal grandfather had spent some of his early years living in Indonesia, and was a small part of the Dutch influence in the country.

We also saw Christian churches including the Catholic cathedral and main Protestant facility. This was a sign of religious tolerance in the country.

After a quick tour of the commercial centre, we headed to our designated accommodation, which was our host's second home. Initially, I was surprised at how modern the house was, however I should not have been surprised, as our hosts were leading members of the medical profession in Semarang. It was contrary to my previous expectations of the quality of housing based on my perceptions and images of housing types common to a developing country.

At this point, however, Fabiola and I were unaware that we were going to reside in accommodation not in the homes of our hosts, and we were going to be living by ourselves with no contact with anyone local. We had understood that we would be billeted with host families, and this would in turn provide the appropriate security. Suddenly we were left alone to fend for ourselves and this was compounded by the fact that we did not speak the language.

The overriding concern was the possibility of something unforeseen happening, with no one we could immediately turn to for assistance. This could range from the loss of electrical power, to a health problem, the latter being worrisome for me. Having said all this, the saving grace was that as mature-aged students with some relevant life experiences, we had the capacity to cope quite adequately.

In the end, Fabiola and I concluded that we could weather any situation and were confident that we would be fine and secure. Overall, we were glad to learn that the rest of the students, who were mostly younger, were all staying in the homes of their respective host families.

Our accommodation was a two-bedroom, double-storey dwelling, and looked very similar to a small Australian townhouse. I occupied the ground floor bedroom so that I could be close to the bathroom. Although the toilet and bathroom were modern, the set-up was consistent with Islamic culture in that the shower recess did not have a shower head, but a cubicle with a trough and a bucket which you used to pour water over yourself.

I felt particularly uncomfortable using the bucket because of the stoma, choosing instead to use the shower, which strangely enough was available outside the cubicle. Personally, I felt that using the shower and the constant flow of water was much easier, but this caused further problems because the water would spread over the rest of the bathroom floor making the whole area very wet. As Fabiola also chose to use the shower outside the cubicle, the problem was further exacerbated, making the clean-up time consuming. I wonder what the locals thought of our bathing practices?

Although there was no hot water, this was not a problem. It was different, but very manageable given the warmer climate. Again, while it was a contrast from what we have in Australia, the situation did not present any major difficulties.

Day one of the study program was almost upon the group. Across the student cohort there was a palpable mixture of nerves and excitement as the representatives from QUT and the tour organisers took the team through our itinerary.

The opportunities offered by the program were indeed challenging, as the plan was for the team to visit nursing academies, polytechnic schools, local hospitals, community health centres and local villages. As well, we were scheduled to visit local projects associated with infection control.

For most of us, this was truly going to be an eye-opening experience. To see and experience this culture and its differences was going to be a valuable, and indeed, a humbling experience for all involved in the program.

Chapter 11

Semarang: A Brief Insight

To be able to smile in the face of emotionally challenging events and stay calm in moments of stress is an ability that everyone can learn.

— Dr Favardin Daliri

Our normal day in the program generally involved a visit to one of the main hospitals in Semarang. As well, visits were made to one or more of the district community health centres known as *Puskesmas,* their sub-centres *Puskesmas Pembantu* and the local support level centres known as *Posyandu.*

This created a very hectic schedule, as the community facilities were scattered over the district with the time allocated to each visit often restricted. Thus, the day was jam-packed with activity, with shortish lunch breaks and limited capacity to attend to personal needs.

For me, the day started with a set routine to ensure that the stoma was as far as possible free from infection. It is worth restating that for an ostomate this is critical as poor care and maintenance can lead to an infection of the wound. As the local tap water was a likely source of infection, I never used it as a cleaning agent. I used only bottled water.

The routine was simply a small adjustment from the usual morning routine in Australia. At home I would remove all the devices during the morning shower; however, in Semarang the bag would still remain attached to the stoma while washing. After the shower I would then detach the bag exposing the stoma, and then wash it with bottled water. The rest of the procedures were as normal including changing the bag, and reattaching it to the stoma ready for the day ahead. I performed a similar routine at the end of the day before retiring for the night.

I made sure that there were always adequate supplies of bottled water in my carry bag while visiting hospitals and health centres. Changing the bag on tour was not a preferred option, as the conditions of the toilets and bathrooms at most of the locations were sub-standard in cleanliness. Therefore, while on the move, and to avoid the risk of infection, attention to the stoma was limited to only draining the bag as necessary, rather than changing it and washing the device. Thankfully, this routine served me well, and I was able to undertake the program of visits and general field activities without requiring any cleaning of the stoma or bag change.

Food intake also became a very important consideration because gastro is to be avoided and the resultant diarrhea and vomiting. People familiar with the workings of a stoma will be aware that this can result in serious consequences due to severe dehydration because of the rapid loss of fluids from the small bowel into the bag. With gastro, I personally tend to lose fluids quickly leading to the loss of vital body salts, which has had an adverse impact on my body. I had gastro on two occasions, which resulted in severe dehydration and hospitalisation. With the information on hand about the difficulties that I would face in the event of a gastro episode while in Indonesia, I took every step to avoid one. Thus, I took special care about the food I ate. I started the day by having a simple basic breakfast of toast and cereal provided by our hosts.

At the lunch breaks, I restricted my food intake to light offerings of sandwiches or biscuits rather that a full hot lunch that included many of the local delights. At dinner we always ate at good quality restaurants, thanks to the host families. While these restaurants looked like safe places to eat, I remained careful, avoiding highly spiced food, and instead preferring to choose a variety of bland dishes.

My advice for ostomates is to set some strict standards that will sustain good health for the digestive system. Looking back, I am pleased to report the fact that in my time spent overseas there were no bouts of gastro, or other stomach- or bowel-related ailments. This was unlike some of my other colleagues on tour who were less careful with the delightful foods on offer, and then had to battle gastro issues during the program. Some of them I believe more than once!

Having established a workable routine to help prevent potential problems relating to the stoma was significant. It gave me the confidence necessary to fully engage in the program and its hectic schedule. From a personal standpoint, being mostly free of any untimely personal health issues was most welcome, as this allowed me to make the most on what would probably be a once-in-a-lifetime experience.

In the first of the visits, we were taken to the Tugurejo and Dr Karadi hospitals, and my first impressions were really quite numbing. To witness the crowded reception area with people lying on the floor, some in apparent distress, and seemingly ignored, was hard to process and took my breath away. This was the first of the humbling experiences encountered throughout the program, and as the days progressed, we saw a health system that would surprise many in Australia. It is characterised in the main from a lack of resources resulting in poor and inadequate facilities and limited delivery of medical services.

There were many impressions of life in Semarang, but one that stood out most was the level of poverty. During my outings I was able to see the hardship felt by many in large parts of the countryside, and the substandard housing these people lived in. However, one must admire the unwavering efforts of the medical staff in meeting the needs of the poor in very difficult circumstances. During my time in Semarang, I met some of the medical people, and in my opinion, the dedication that these people showed in working with the sick could not be faulted.

The issue that particularly caught my attention was the absence of proper procedures in the prevention of cross infection. While there was no doubt that nurses and other health care workers in the system were knowledgeable of the broader principles of hygiene, the actual practice, due to the lack of resources, was different. As an ostomate and one conscious about infection, I observed that a common practice was to use the same syringe to insert antibiotics into the intravenous tubing of patients. Alarmingly, these procedures were also undertaken without the use of gloves and protective clothing. It was also visible that in both hospitals and community health centres, nursing and other health staff were accustomed to wearing open footwear as opposed to shoes, which is contrary to basic standards in preventing cross-infection.

I learned that the needles and syringes were reused due to inadequate supplies. More disturbingly, this reuse of basic medical equipment was also driven by the need to minimise costs for families, as a high proportion were poor.

This was all very distressing given that prevention of cross-infection is central to my physical wellbeing. In every sense I lamented this situation, and felt very concerned for the local people who had similar medical problems to mine, and the risks and hardships they faced and had to overcome. However, it was obvious that these realities did not deter the doctors, nurses and support staff in their endeavours to provide the best medical aid to patients.

Most of all, special tribute must be paid to the young nurses, and in our visits to the hospitals and community centres, special time was always set aside to spend time with this group, acknowledging the common bond between nurses. These girls were very different from us: all wore head scarves following the Islamic faith. Yet nationality, culture, religion and language were no barriers to enjoying each other's company and sharing the usual nursing banter.

Unfortunately, due to limited time in a hectic program, I was not able to come into contact with patients with ostomies, and therefore unable to observe the treatment methods used for these patients. I was, however, able to talk about the importance of wound care with the nurses, in the hope that some of my knowledge and experience could be used when treating this medical condition.

After engaging in, and observing, all the activities required by the program, it was now time to say goodbye to our medical colleagues and return home. It was also a moment to reflect somewhat sadly on the realities of the communities around Semarang, and be thankful that I had the chance to observe and to understand the struggles they endure. While looking forward to returning home, there was a tinge of sadness about leaving many of the wonderful people that I had met.

As a lifelong learning exercise, the trip was worthwhile. In our development as professional nurses, the program took us out of our comfort zone to a place where health care provision was so different from and alien to our senses. Its value lay in the opportunity to understand and believe, that irrespective of prevailing adverse conditions, adaption and commitment by the individual remain the most important ingredients in the work and life of the caregiver. This experience has resonated throughout my nursing career, giving me the capacity to rise to the occasion, and use some of the knowledge gained to enhance the lives of others less fortunate.

In reflecting on this experience overseas, this new understanding of life in a different country has given me a real appreciation of how lucky I am with the level of medical support available in Australia.

From the outset, the overriding concern in travelling to Indonesia was the question about my health and the potential risks associated with having a stoma.

In highlighting the ground-breaking elements of this trip, it is worth mentioning that the previous trip to Canada followed a temporary ileostomy, which tested the resilience of the stoma under different conditions. In this trip to Indonesia, I had a permanent ileostomy (total removal of the large bowel). This was a much different set of circumstances altogether. So, while there was some confidence from the success of the previous trip, this visit to Indonesia was new territory.

Happy to say, there were no hitches. With the day-to-day experiences and remedial measures taken, I learned things about myself, especially when it came to managing my health outside the security of my country.

This outcome was important and was a time for much euphoria at being able to survive another overseas trip without any hitches. Importantly, this outcome was the next big step in the quest to live a normal life and further entrenched my confidence in remaining health safe while travelling overseas.

The successful outcome of this visit to Indonesia was testimony to the fact that for an ostomate most of these overseas adventures are well within reach, provided appropriate due diligence is taken to ensure all care is taken and all unexpected contingencies addressed.

I believe strongly that the methods adopted to prevent or avert infection played a very large part in ensuring the success of the trip. In particular, the diligence associated with bathing and adhering to strict procedures in cleaning the stoma using safe water.

An important point to remember is that when in doubt always default to bottled water or other secure alternatives. Even in developed countries potable water can be unsafe, so use bottled water to clean the stoma.

Do not take chances!

As mentioned previously, it is important to be careful with food. In Semarang I took special care in the choice of food and this must have paid off, as I totally avoided stomach upsets. Again, it is worth reiterating that the priority always is to avoid any unnecessary medical treatment while overseas.

Therefore, to my ostomy, colectomy and other similar friends, the lesson here is that you are not at all restricted in travelling and the enjoyment it brings. Go for it!

Chapter 12

The Finishing Line

However mean your life is, meet it and live it; do not shun and call it hard names. It looks poorest when you are richest.
— Henry David Thoreau

Back home in Australia after completing the program in Indonesia, it was time to tackle the final stages of the nursing degree and complete the course by the end of the semester, which ended in July 2015. Like most students hoping to graduate, there was apprehension about gaining work in a hospital as employment for graduates was not guaranteed. All students knew this, even going back to the early days of the course, as there were limited positions. Given this situation, the best response for a student nurse, was to focus on academic accomplishments, essentially achieving a high GPA (Grade Point Average) across the three years of study. In most instances, a high grade would assist in securing employment in a city hospital, whereas something lower could result in being appointed as a nurse in a rural location. Such an outcome was not exactly palatable given my husband's employment was based in Brisbane.

Fortunately, I had already achieved a high GPA, and knowing

the ultimate grading would now rest on two heavily weighted assignments, all my efforts were directed towards ensuring that they were completed extremely well.

Another essential requirement to complete the degree involved the mandatory completion of practical assessments in a hospital environment. The first of these was at the Lady Cilento Children's Hospital in the southside of the city, working in a medical ward for four weeks. The next rotation was at The Wesley Hospital with an assignment in the emergency centre, also for a four-week period. Both practical rotations provided the opportunity to be at the coalface of patient care. In regard to The Wesley, there was a sense of gratitude for the care given me over such an extended period, and therefore I was very keen to secure a position here as a way of paying back all that had been done for me.

While encountering the stresses associated with completing the course, I was further affected by the death of my paternal grandmother. This greatly saddened me because more than anything else it was my intent that she would witness my graduation as a nurse. From my discussions with her, I know she would have been most proud of my achievements, and it was thus very upsetting that she was not going to be around when this occurred.

As with all the student cohort, we moved along the pathway leading to the end of the course, and on completing all the assessments, it was time to sit back and wait for the results. I can distinctly recall the high level of nervousness while scanning the computer daily. And then they came. This was a special moment in my life. I had graduated with a GPA of 6.7 and placed within the top five per cent of all students. Adding to this was also the sixth consecutive dean's commendation, and with this an invitation to join the university's Golden Key Honours Society for academic excellence.

I was so elated. My key goals had been achieved. The only thing left was to get a job, and surely these results would increase the chances of securing a position, possibly quite quickly. It was time to find out.

As is the norm, I registered with Job Search via the usual online portals and waited eagerly for notifications and alerts on the availability of vacant graduate positions at hospitals.

As if by providence, I received a notification from The Wesley Hospital regarding a program for graduate nurses. This was really exciting, as it would be fantastic to work alongside my mother, and continue the next generation of nurses in our family to work for Uniting Health.

So, brimming with confidence, I fronted to the interview and immersed myself in the recruitment process, knowing full well that psychometric testing would be a key component of the selection process. To prepare I practised at home using examples of these tests to become more acquainted with the formats used. The selection process was indeed quite gruelling, and true to form, the psychometric test was quite difficult. At its conclusion, I felt that my results would be below standard.

Another part of the selection process involved participation in a group interview, and I was confident in performing well given my life experience and knowledge acquired after ten years in the airline environment. This was not to be. In reality, there was no excuse in not excelling in this opportunity to display my skill sets, but somehow, I became distracted, and my performance was again well below par. At the end of the selection process, there was a feeling of being flat because of the disappointment at my overall presentation.

Despite my performance at the interview, there was still some hope that my strong academic record would find a way through. However, shortly after the interview, the hospital notified me that I was unsuccessful. This was devasting news! Almost immediately negative doubts began to creep in, including thoughts that by not securing a position with The Wesley, then there was also the likelihood of not winning a position elsewhere. I found myself sitting on the sofa in tears, and this was not helped when I found out that a friend of mine who had presented at the same interview had been successful, and would commence placement shortly.

Shaking off the initial disappointment, I repeated this process at The Wesley when additional positions became available, and also at some other private hospitals, but again with no success. A placement now seemed too far away. With the continuing lack of success, there was this massive struggle in coming to terms with the unfolding situation, particularly given my maturity and academic achievements. It all did not make sense, especially the frustration knowing that some twenty students who were part of my cohort had already secured employment ahead of me.

I had no option but to persist, and an opportunity became available at the Prince Charles Hospital in the north of Brisbane. This public facility took a somewhat different approach from that of the private sector hospitals. Applicants were required to respond via an online portal, answering some basic questions, then attach a cover letter and a CV. For the first time, I felt more comfortable in the simplicity of the process, as it seemed that the organisation was trying to gauge a preliminary appraisal of my strengths up front. My application was followed quickly by an invitation to an interview to be held over the following weeks.

Adamant not to miss out this time around, I set about nailing this opportunity by undertaking research that would enhance my position at the interview. In gathering as much information as possible, I made every effort to contact people familiar with the hospital, and in doing so, learned some useful clues on hospital operations as well as its organisational culture. Adding to this mix, I spent much time and endeavour delving into specific areas, hoping to have an edge.

The recruitment process of Queensland Health was easier to negotiate, appropriately targeted, and generally more akin to my expectations. To gauge the appropriate skill of an individual, the evaluative process was directly tied towards the clinical aspects of nursing, and linked directly to the ward. In this setting, there were searching questions testing knowledge on a range of medical issues which I comfortably answered. Overall, I had a feeling of relief knowing that my responses were concise and eloquent, and that my performance on the day was good.

I was confident of a favourable outcome, and in the space of twenty-four hours I was notified that I had secured a position. Making me more pleased was the feedback that in the process of selection I had performed at a very high standard.

While I was excited about my success, I also felt some unease when told that that the position was in the cardio-thoracic ward. My main concern stemmed from my lack of knowledge in this area, given that throughout the nursing course there was never any exposure to cardiac nursing, and as a student I had never undertaken any practical work or assessments in this area.

Following the usual protocols attached to a job offer by Queensland Health, I had to respond within twenty-four hours. I tried to objectively assess the situation, as the offer was not exactly my preference, and I discussed the matter at length with my sister who was employed by Queensland Health, my husband and parents. In the end, albeit with some reluctance, I accepted the offer, as nursing appointments for graduates were hard to secure, and to decline was not a good option as other opportunities could be scarce further down the track.

It has always been my belief that life has its twist and turns and this can often be quite uncanny. Having accepted the position as a stepping stone to the next phase, unexpectedly, there was a turn in events. Just prior to confirming my acceptance, I received a phone message from a highly embarrassed Queensland Health representative advising that there had been some kind of clerical error, and that the position on offer actually did not exist. In one way this had let me off the hook, but on the other, I was concerned that the placement and indeed employment opportunity were in jeopardy. However, to my relief I was told that as a position had already been offered as a result of the interview, an alternative placement would be found in an area that was of interest to me. Without any hesitation I chose the general surgical ward at The Prince Charles Hospital.

Always believing that events of this nature happen for a reason, and usually for the better, I had now landed my area of choice. Importantly for me, this was the opportunity to access stoma patients and to interact closely with the wound and stoma team.

This was a great outcome as a platform was now in place that I could realise my desire to interact with and assist patients living with stomas and similar types of medical conditions. I was ecstatic, as this small but important step placed me directly in stoma therapy care, and I was mindful also that this could be the catalyst for more doors to open in this area.

Initially, the general surgical ward I worked in was part of a combined ward incorporating general surgical, thoracic, vascular and urology. However, midway through 2017, the ward was split into two areas: general surgical in one area, and thoracic, vascular and urology in the other. I chose to remain in the general surgical area, stepping into a twenty-eight-bed ward with the ratio of one nurse to every four patients, and nurses working together in teams.

Taking a proactive stance, I approached the unit manager in an effort to gain more experience in wound care. My initiative was well received. After discussions, a broad-based agreement was established for me to undertake six eight-week shifts acting as a replacement for staff members who were on secondment, or on leave. I was elated at such a positive response, but at the same time aware that this exercise was going to be quite challenging, as I still had to complete my contracted hours on the ward. That made the additional workloads quite tiring, although very rewarding.

As I got more involved, I discovered that building relationships with patients relatively easy, especially being able to relate to many of these people at different levels. In particular I found my lived experience was an asset, and at this point the capacity to discuss and personalise life with a stoma in my interactions with patients was very rewarding. Also, it was not unusual for me to receive a request from the wound and stoma team to assist with a patient wanting to discuss matters after an ileostomy or similar type surgery. So, even with these small steps, there was sufficient encouragement in my role for me to believe I was on the correct path to become an advocate and to assist people with bowel disorders.

Now feeling satisfied working as a nurse with a focus on stoma recipients, it was also very heartening when witnessing a turnaround in the attitude of patients, especially knowing my small part in creating this change. So, as a result of the many unforgettable encounters with patients, I was already blessed with these rewards, even in the early days of the nursing career.

Most of all, I recollect being told by so many people that I was where I needed to be. These words ring true even to this very moment. As in my first Virgin Airlines moment, I had again arrived in a space where I should be, and wanted to be, and that I was now in the best workplace possible.

Firstly, the current public hospital environment provides much support for new graduates with clinical nurse teachers available every day of the week to consult over matters that are not well understood. As well, mandating ratios of 1:4 or 2:8 between patients and nurses offers much assistance in effectively managing workloads, and for new graduates it is very beneficial for learning on the job.

Secondly, the stoma team at Prince Charles recognised very early that, as a person with lived experience, I could be used as a good resource. This in turn has allowed me to grow in skills and confidence in resolving practical issues associated with stoma patients, and consequently become a developing asset.

In utilising this lived experience another door was opened with an invitation from the wound and stoma team to present my story at education days and seminars conducted at the hospital. These were in-house forums allowing me to address attendees from the perspective of someone living with the condition, and thus convey and present an existing patient's experience for the benefit of medical staff. Importantly in these new initiatives, I got the opportunity to meet other clinicians and invitees from ostomy groups and private companies with a commercial interest in the manufacture and retailing of ostomy and related products. My exposure to these groups while not directly affiliated with the hospital was yet another step forward, underscored by coming into contact with The Australian Council for Stoma Associations Inc., and in the commercial scene, Liberty Medical. In a positive move, both of these agencies expressed much interest in engaging my services in speaking engagements outside the formal hospital environment.

As these interrelationships blossomed, interest was generated in other medical circles, leading the wound care department of the hospital to invite me to participate in and present my story at their regular wound care days. Adding to further recognition was the publication of articles that I wrote in the staff newsletter and other platforms, highlighting and showcasing my advocacy and skills in stoma care.

Regarding my physical capacity to cope with the rigours of working intensively with patients, it is worth mentioning that the existence of my stoma was in no way different from my last years at Virgin Airlines after I underwent the ileostomy. Admittedly in this new role there were some instances of minor troubles on the ward, with the occasional bag leak while on shift. By and large these issues were easily rectified without any noticeable interruption to the working day.

As a stoma patient, a matter to be considered carefully when working in a hospital ward is the issue of infection. A gastro infection is common and very confronting as it can lead to a serious health risk.

Generally speaking, whether in the community or in a hospital, risk awareness is most important, because the consequences of gastro and its unpleasant symptoms can be debilitating. As mentioned earlier, the impact of infection can vary between individuals, and in my experience a gastro attack usually leads to severe dehydration, and in one instance even a minor kidney malfunction. I can vividly recall that in one year, three out of four of my hospital admissions were directly due to gastro, when there was the urgent need to be treated with several bags of IV fluids as a precaution against severe dehydration.

Therefore, when it was feared that my health might be compromised due to an infection in the ward, the team leaders at the hospital have been professionally diligent in allowing me to change my designated allocation of work. Undoubtedly this intervention by managers and team leaders has allowed me to avert the problem, and I am truly grateful for their duty of care in making my life much less traumatic.

My employment at Prince Charles was further secured when I was offered a permanent position after I completed my graduate year.

With this added security under my belt, a new chapter of life began to unfold as I started contemplating starting a family. Under the circumstances, this was a big decision as it was uncertain if the pregnancy and its resultant side effects would have any adverse impacts on my body. It was indeed uncharted territory in respect to the risks involved. For example, it was unclear how pregnancy would affect my nutritional levels given that with only a small intestine, being pregnant could require the consumption of other and therefore different foods for their nutritional value to care for the foetus, while at the same time ensuring the proper operation of the stoma. This was a real concern, as following the ileostomy there were a number of instances of lack of energy because of poor nutritional intake. So, the issue centred firstly on nutrition for the development of the foetus, and secondly, on my capacity to carry the pregnancy for the full term.

To overcome some of these concerns I consulted a gynaecologist and the usual rounds of testing were undertaken including scans, blood tests and ovarian reserve tests. Happily, all the results were normal with the specialist saying that from his perspective he could see no medical reason for my body not being able to conceive naturally. Also, the colorectal surgeon was comfortable with the decision.

Happily, within two months, I became pregnant with the child to be born in late December 2017. There was much elation with this outcome, and like any expectant mother I set about preparing for the new arrival.

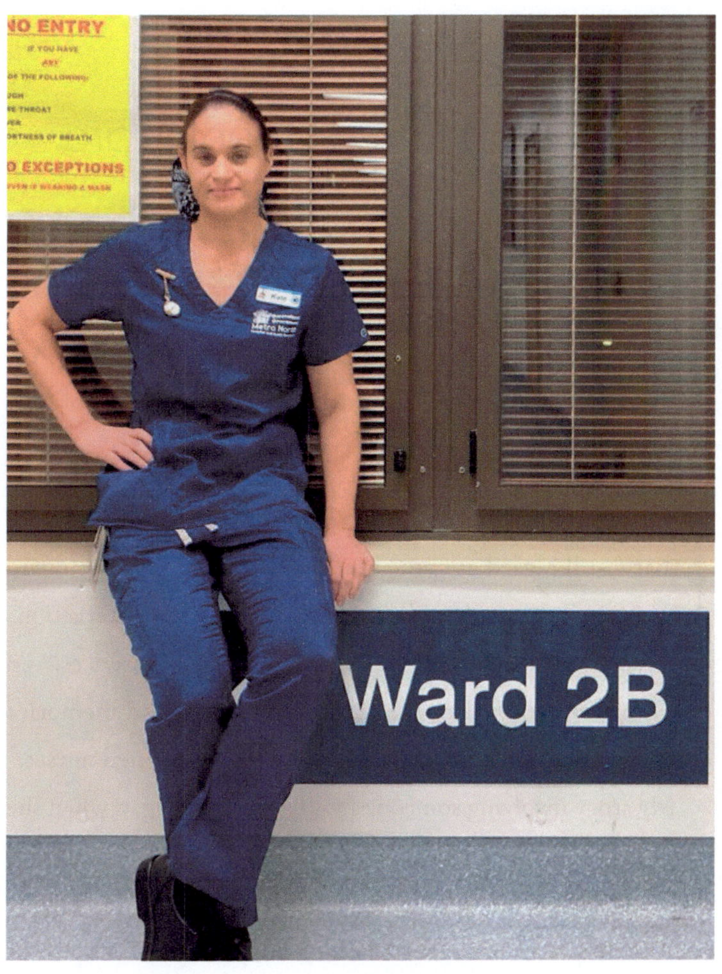

Embracing my work at the Prince Charles Hospital in Brisbane

Chapter 13

An Insight into Patient Care

Kindness can transform someone's dark moment into a blaze of light. You'll never know how much your caring matters. Make a difference.

— **Amy Leigh Mercree**

In the early days working on the wards, I recall two instances that I still regard as special moments, which I would like to share with the reader. I hope that describing my interactions will resonate with those who have had similar experiences, and that these stories will awaken the reservoir of good memories about the care given by the many wonderful, dedicated nurses.

My story involving someone I will call Anne began when she was a patient at The Prince Charles Hospital. Anne, who was suffering from ulcerative colitis disease, had recently undergone an ileostomy. As she was only twenty-five years old, the idea of a stoma was extremely confronting for a person so young.

Therefore, when I was assigned to Anne, I approached my task with some trepidation having had an ileostomy at the age of thirty-one, and remembering the extent of my emotional turmoil. Knowing the importance of relating carefully to her situation, I used my experience all those years ago as a patient immediately after the ileostomy, as the basis of my discussions with Anne. I recalled in great detail how the nurses supported me, utilising their skills and compassion, thus giving me a better appreciation and understanding of the reality of the situation. Especially, I remembered the tireless work to bring clarity in dealing with the range of confronting issues, and how this brought comfort to strengthen my resolve and to move forward with greater conviction.

Thus, fully armed with these memories, I walked into Anne's room for the first time after her surgery. Looking into her eyes I could see her anguish and despair, and at that particular moment my memories came flooding back. At our first contact, it was clear the process of repair would be slow, and hence the need to be mindful and cautious in respecting her feelings and the level of emotions she displayed.

As we talked, I started by adopting the normal approach embedded in the training of nurses, which was to provide support, comfort and reassurance to the patient. So, with Anne, as with any patient in my care, I first asked about her health generally, and then slowly moved to the stoma by asking salient questions about physical discomfort and particular medical concerns that she was having as a result of the surgery. In gauging her position as best possible, I shifted the conversation to the management of wound care, by emphasising the significance of good practices in attending to the stoma as an essential element in her daily life. In particular I highlighted the importance of a healthy stoma in preventing setbacks to her lifestyle, and the high probability that normality could be attained, while accepting that life at that juncture for her looked very difficult.

For Anne, as in any young person experiencing such a dramatic transformation, reassurances given at the time were all well and good, however, the idea of having a waste bag attached to the body is not something that one can easily comprehend or become accustomed to. The common and persisting worry about a waste bag that affects many stoma patients, especially at the outset, is the belief that the device is contrary to everything that is normal for any person, let alone a young adult.

Aside from the waste bag, for Anne the usual fears were already in play and these included similar questions that I had encountered as some of the key challenges ahead. As a reminder, these included the capacity of being able to dress well, relationships with others, especially with the opposite sex, being pregnant and having children, social acceptance and stigmas, and of course the management of day-to-day living with a stoma.

I made every effort to reinforce the fact that the apparent disability of a stoma was in fact not a disability but rather a distraction. I introduced this level of reinforcement in a rational and calm manner embedded within a framework citing the many positive experiences of other stoma patients. Then, actually revealing myself as a stoma patient brought much relief, followed by an increasing belief that the messaging was indeed authentic, and hopefully leading to a higher level of acceptance.

One of the most pressing and widely endemic concerns among ileostomy patients is physical presentation. The belief among many ostomates, particularly the younger set, is that the stoma and waste bag are extremely visible devices because of their apparent bulkiness, which restrict the choice of clothing. In taking this further, the enduring sentiment in the case of a woman or younger girl is that their only dress choice would be limited to baggy clothing or other loose-fitting garments to hide the bag. In talking through some of my patients' problems regarding personal presentation, which is a cause of much anxiety, we were able to discuss openly the minimal problems I personally encountered in this area. Here the emphasis was on the wide range of choices available, without any regard to awkwardness. In essence, it was a fact that the idea of only reverting to baggy clothing was long gone and within reason body-fitting clothing was *still the go*. Hence, in the ensuing conversation, and by way of personal experience, I was able to reinforce the fact that there were few limitations to dressing in the daily choice of clothing, and to debunk the view of imaginary personal restrictions.

Speaking for myself, the only garment I miss wearing is the cheong sum. Women of Asian heritage who wear this dress would know exactly what I am talking about. Even so, I believe that wearing this garment is still possible. Apart from this, and a few other examples, there are hardly any clothes that a stoma patient cannot wear.

Recalling my own earlier fears in this direction, it became clear how unfortunate this reaction was, but at the time there was limited knowledge and awareness regarding the current and developing improvements in bag technology. Like Anne, this perception by patients when first faced with the prospect of a stoma is mostly about a waste bag looking very much like a bubble on the waistline.

In countering this false perception, it is worth dwelling briefly on the remarkable improvements in bag technology and supporting devices that have developed over the years. They have improved from awkward-sized bags to slim replacements better designed to fit the body, and generally almost undetectable under clothing. As well, these new designs are more efficient in their operation and therefore very user-friendly, particularly in relation to removal and reattachment.

When discussing matters of concern with patients, the conversation invariably returns to the question of social acceptance, already mentioned in Chapter 5. This is a critical issue felt across both genders, and while my discussions to date seems to be focused on the female side of the equation, it is also necessary to point out that this trauma is also felt by men. Perhaps this is experienced in different ways in men, but for them, life can be equally as difficult when faced with changes in lifestyle after having an ileostomy, colostomy or similar.

I believe that deflecting the negative perceptions surrounding social acceptance is important when discussing patients' concerns about having a stoma. To a significant extent it is the fear of the unknown that is the driving force here. Without understanding the reality of what actually occurs, the negative view will mostly prevail unless effectively counteracted. This is certainly a futile way of thinking, but one that can be easily corrected

In talking with Anne, I noted that she was particularly traumatised by the challenges of being socially accepted, and therefore it also became necessary to try to relieve some of those anxieties. We started to examine how social acceptance actually occurred in real life. I described the experiences of my thirteen years spent as a member of ground staff at Virgin Airlines, focusing mainly on the last three years there after having the ileostomy. The point I made was that in all circumstances and at all times, I never felt any different from my fellow workers even though I was saddled with a stoma. More importantly, it was my general belief that the stoma was never perceived as being odd by my peers. This was supported by the fact that it did not restrict my choice of dress, how I looked and behaved, and did not in any way impinge on my ability to perform my work.

I have found that people in society are in the main oblivious to someone having an ileostomy, colostomy or urostomy. I strongly believe that ostomates can in fact be very relaxed about being socially accepted. To this end, we must be thankful to the societal and related positive changes that have occurred around education, understanding and empathy. This, in turn, has engendered the trend to high levels of acceptance, and understanding of the individual no matter their circumstances.

While not wishing to labour this point, it is important to again acknowledge the work of many in this area, including the tireless efforts of Jessica Grossman, a person of great inspiration. To witness her courage and success in educating the community about the normality of a person with a bowel condition is an encouragement for an ostomate to believe in her words that 'there is no need to hide your situation as you are as normal as anyone else'.

Along with this concern about social acceptance is also the constant management of the stoma, involving changing and cleaning the bag. The main concern here is how to avoid accidents and a malfunction of the system leading to leaks and other not-so-desirable misadventures. Altogether, these are frightful thoughts for many who live with an ileostomy, colostomy or something similar. In helping Anne, I was able to use my personal experience to advise the best ways of caring for the stoma, and minimising leakages and other accidents.

For an ostomate, the best outcomes are attained through a trial-and-error basis, just as I experienced after having a number of accidents, particularly in the early days after the surgery. In this way, individuals will develop the ability to better manage the system more effectively and to their personal benefit. However, and irrespective of all the positive assurances given, it is always important to point out that there is never a guarantee that accidents will not occur. However, the comforting thought is that they can be controlled and normal activity can be resumed quickly.

So, in nursing Anne, we developed a good rapport and even friendship, always combining the serious side of the medical condition with an interspersion of jokes about the stoma. For all those familiar with the workings of an ileostomy, these people will understand that when waste is discharged into the bag, there is quite often a gurgle or weird sounds which, to those nearby, would sound somewhat like a fart. We would both have a good laugh at this, particularly in looking at the faces of people when these noises occur. To us, the wearers of bags, these events are normal, however to almost everyone else this is quite often a little bit embarrassing, as they are unaware as to exactly what lies under our garments.

At the time of writing this book, I am aware that Anne is now well into a happy, normal life with a long-term partner, having adapted to the changes that have occurred to her. Importantly from Anne's standpoint, the surgery has given her a new lease in life without the constant pain and discomfort common to many ulcerative colitis disease sufferers. It might be difficult for those who have not had bowel problems to understand this fully, but in reality, an ileostomy can in most circumstances be appreciated as a gift that ultimately allows a person to live a full and fruitful life, a position that is generally not achievable otherwise.

Anne and I still keep in contact, and I am really happy to see that she continues to travel well. From time to time, we meet with a trip to the movies, always challenging each other as to whose bag is going to burst and what this is going to do to the whole theatre if it does.

Overall, being able to assist patients to make things happen, and to make a difference is so rewarding. In my daily working life, there is much satisfaction from the opportunities I have to assist those in need of support and care, and for this, I remain very grateful.

Always in my memory is a more elderly gentleman whom I will call Bill, diagnosed with bowel cancer and who was fitted with a colostomy bag following surgery. For most people, having such a device attached to the body is very traumatic no matter whether one is as young as Anne, or a much older person like Bill. In fact, their reactions and concerns are generally very similar.

To put Bill's concerns into perspective, he saw his colostomy as a dreadful impediment, as his appendage, although lifesaving, was fitted further down the bowel tract. This makes the waste much more difficult to manage than an ileostomy, which connects directly from the small intestine to the bag. More specifically, in the case of an ileostomy, the digested food and subsequent waste does not travel down the large bowel, and therefore the output or body waste is very much different and best described as lighter than that from a colostomy.

Even from the perspective of an ostomy patient, it is easier to understand that having a colostomy is potentially harder to accept because of the dramatic change in how the body functions and impacts on lifestyle. In a cumulative sense, when adding the usual concerns, a colostomy can in fact be sometimes seen as a bridge too far to cross.

And so, when I was first assigned to nurse Bill, it was clear that he was undergoing a very difficult adjustment in coming to grips with his problems. Therefore, softening the impact and somehow breaching the barrier of trying to calm his fears was going to be a hard task. Clearly there was no silver bullet readily available except to resort to professionalism, personal experience, empathy and patience.

Being well into my training with newly attained skills and more experience, I was more competent in explaining in detail many aspects about wound care, including some of the more intricate ways of managing a colostomy. The central focus again was to provide a platform to minimise accidents to the extent that the patient could be less fearful of this occurring in public spaces. Getting to this point is very much a confidence matter on the part of the individual, and I believe nurses can engage in this role as a crucial phase when caring for patients with a colostomy. Witnessing the improvement in patients when they gain more confidence in managing their situation is very rewarding, as it was in the case of Bill and others in my care.

Looking back on my encounter with Bill, we achieved a lot in conversations, leaving me with the feeling that these discussions may have acted as the stimulus for him to move forward, irrespective of the apparent setbacks. Importantly, it was most pleasing to see him accepting that his condition was not in an absolutely irretrievable situation, as he had earlier thought. There was now a good chance that over time his outlook will shift to a more positive tack. I was somewhat sad to say goodbye to him on the day that he left hospital, but was also pleased about my small part in assisting him in the next step on his journey.

As well as Bill, I have nursed many patients recovering from various bowel surgeries and that has been most rewarding, not only regarding helping to manage their challenges, but also to witness the sense of relief as they realise that there is light at the end of the tunnel. Being part of such a rewarding activity has given me much pleasure.

It must be said, however, that working with these patients is not always a one-way street, as I have gained professionally from these encounters. This is consistent with my pursuit to learn as much as possible about the medical complexities associated with bowel diseases. Importantly, these experiences have provided invaluable currency on a wide array of medical issues that I would not have been exposed to otherwise. Furthermore, in engaging with these patients, I was more motivated to continue research and investigations into a wide range of data relating to diseases of the bowel, their anatomical implications, and to critically review medical interventions and their impacts after surgery.

Chapter 14

Off Hospitals and Surgeries

The greatest glory in living lies not in never falling but in rising every time we fall.

— **Nelson Mandela**

At about 3:30 am on 14 July 2017 in the middle of a night shift, after I had just finished transfusing a patient and was about to begin the usual rounds of routine observations, I started to feel a little unwell with abdominal pain. Trying to dismiss this as possibly a slight touch of gastro which was around at the time, I continued working, but the pain persisted, quickly intensifying into bouts of nausea. By the end of the shift, I had deteriorated to the point where I began to vomit frequently and was concerned. The pain seemed most unusual, especially as I had been mostly free from pain and discomfort since the colectomy.

Little did I know that in front of me was the start of a traumatic period beyond anything experienced before. By every measure, the health problems of the past seventeen years now paled into insignificance, as I was unknowingly on the cusp of fighting to save my life. And that of my unborn child.

Somehow, while increasingly being overcome by pain and nausea, I was able to complete my handover of patients to the incoming shift. As soon as this was finalised, I presented to the emergency clinic at The Holy Spirit Hospital, a private hospital attached to the public facility of my workplace. Having this emergency clinic so close was most fortunate, as I received assistance very quickly, and for the time being quelled the rising and cascading anxieties.

As normal, the initial treatment was consistent with suspected gastroenteritis, no different from my suspicions when first confronted with the pain some five hours earlier. Given the initial pre-diagnosis, I was feeling somewhat relieved, as having had this problem before, it was seemingly not a hassle, and therefore all would soon return to normality.

The full diagnosis was thorough, involving a series of tests and a CT scan, and although it was generally inconclusive, the doctors believed that gastro was probably not the cause, but rather I had an obstruction in the small bowel. As most of the previous treatments for the ongoing bowel condition, including the management of my pregnancy, were managed by specialists attached to The Wesley Hospital, contact was made with my colorectal surgeon and obstetrics team, and I was transferred to their care.

On arrival at The Wesley Hospital, the medical team immediately began treatment for a small bowel obstruction, initially involving a conservative approach with the introduction of clear fluids to clear the bowel. This was then followed by observations of the stoma to determine if it was functioning accordingly. However, there was little or no respite from the pain, which was contrary to the usual response from initial efforts to resolve the partially blocked bowel.

In the next twenty-four hours, the pain progressively worsened, and became almost unbearable. Looking to buy a little more time to allow the initial treatment to work, strong painkillers were administered, but despite this there was little relief from the intense pain. By this time, I was vomiting, and as an option anti-emetic therapy was then administered. Unfortunately, this was also to no avail.

As the situation began to spiral downwards it was beginning to pose a real threat to me, and this was further complicated when the stoma bag showed traces of blood, something that had never occurred before. It started to become even more concerning when it was noticeable the stoma was now a dusky colour, an indication that something unusual and drastic was happening around the wound.

Now more fearful, my thoughts started to turn towards other concerns, thinking perhaps the condition was heading into an advanced stage of septicaemia. In witnessing the visible changes in the performance of the small bowel and the stoma, it was clear that there was serious trouble ahead.

In the early hours of that Saturday, the medicos decided to perform surgery immediately, and I was taken to theatre for an emergency laparotomy. As it was explained to me by the surgeon on call, the problem was suspected to be an intestinal ischemia which generally occurs when blood flowing through the major arteries that supply the small intestine slows or stops.

The condition has many potential causes, however in this case it appeared that the issue was most likely associated with a blockage or a twisting of the bowel, thus restricting blood flow, in turn causing severe abdominal pain and discomfort.

So much was happening now, so much pain and discomfort, so much fear, yet through all this haze while being wheeled into theatre my thoughts were all about the baby. Having a child after undergoing a total colectomy and living with an ileostomy was always going to be a journey into unknown territory. However, everything was moving at a speed denying me the opportunity to seek any form of reassurance or information on this matter from the medical staff, and my husband and family. As events unfolded, and alone in my thoughts and fears about the threat to the baby, these emotions were overwhelming as I succumbed to the anaesthetic.

Awakening from surgery, covered in tubes and feeling very sick and sore, my first reaction was to revert to my last thoughts before going under and that was to enquire about the child. To my relief I was informed that the baby was fine and had not been impacted by the surgery. All was seemingly well at this juncture.

With so much at stake I immediately asked the surgeon for details of the operation, and in particular the causes of the pain, the blood, and the resultant impact on the condition of the stoma. I was subsequently informed that my small intestine had indeed been twisted, resulting in stemming the blood flow and causing all the side effects. In terms of a prognosis, there was a reassurance that the issue had now been rectified by the removal of the twist and straightening out of the bowel, in turn allowing it to perform normally again. Obviously, this news was a welcome relief knowing that while there was still a battle ahead, this hurdle would be overcome by gaining full recovery over the coming weeks. Importantly, the baby was thriving, and there was good reason for a positive outlook that in a short period the pain would disappear, and my life and the pregnancy would continue as normal. As was usual for me, it was time to sit back and work the usual recovery phase.

How wrong I was to think that this would be so simple!

The next twelve hours were possibly one of the scariest times of my life, and something that I never expected to occur because of the apparent good outcome of the recent surgery and prognosis. It started within a few hours after the procedure when I began to feel pain, which was immense and consuming. The best description here is to paint a scene of being totally incapable of sitting in bed for any length of time. I would get on my feet, walk over to the window to take my mind off the pain, and then back to the bed, repeating this action in a continuous pattern. Adding to the concern associated with the deteriorating condition, the medical team was now aware that my respiratory rate was high. My heart rate was 170 beats per minute, and my blood pressure was very low. These were clear signs that something was astray, and medically consistent with the body reacting adversely to a form of severe infection or intolerance.

As I continued to slide downhill, the point was reached when a medical emergency or MERT was called. I was attended by a 'crash' team working to stabilise the highly threatening condition. Being a nurse, I was fully aware that this was very close to a

Code Blue, one step away from a full cardiac arrest. By this time, although semi-conscious because of the pain and drugs administered, I was still able to understand my predicament. I was determined to hang on to life. Everything around me was in a blur while the medicos worked on me, but there was an incident or moment that I will remember for the rest of my life, and it is something worth sharing.

Although brought up as a Christian, I cannot claim to be strongly spiritual in my thinking, however, while being treated by the crash team I can vividly recall a presence close to me at the bedside. In this vision I saw a lady looking down at my face, telling me not to be afraid and reassuring me that all would be well. It is difficult to describe my feelings exactly at that moment, but it is certainly true that even in that current state of mind, those special words of encouragement were of tremendous comfort and strength.

This episode is not something that can be explained easily, and to the sceptic, even believable. However, upon reflection, I am inclined to mention this incident because the episode did have some meaning while I was in so much distress.

Much later during the recovery phase and with a mind free from extreme pain and strong medications, I felt the presence was that of my grandmother who had recently passed away and was there to help, support and protect me through all the traumas. Apart from this brief mention of a particular experience, there is no more to add except to leave it to the discretion of the readers to form their own opinions.

Having been stabilised by the crash team, I was transferred

to theatre for an emergency laparotomy. This time, although heavily sedated and in a sub-conscious state, there was still an acute awareness that undoubtedly my life and that of the baby were in grave danger. There was nothing left now other than to succumb to the surgery and the outcomes and eventualities, good or bad, that lay ahead: all of which were beyond my control.

I was extremely fearful of a grim outcome because of the physical impacts of undergoing two emergency surgeries in barely twenty-four hours. It was also a crucial time where, if my survival became a major risk, it would be up to my husband with the support of my family to make key decisions to ensure my wellbeing. All was now left in the hands of my surgeon and my obstetrician to make the right decision, even if it might also be difficult for them.

From a medical perspective, the critical issue was the decisions to be made if my life was threatened. Although this was never openly discussed, it was always on the cards that if the surgeon and obstetrician felt my survival would necessitate the termination of the pregnancy, then this option would be taken.

Clearly, any decision would be made in consultation with the surgeon, the obstetrician, my husband and family. It was indeed a heavy burden for all concerned to carry. Undoubtedly, for the specialists assisting me, to my husband and parents, this was a confronting situation, and one that was not expected given the apparent success of the first procedure less than twenty-four hours earlier. Therefore, no one in the family group was mentally or emotionally prepared to address or weigh up all the issues and impacts, and to come to a decision on my behalf. As I faced an anaesthetic for the second time, it was impossible for me to gauge their anxieties, and it was only much later in my recovery that I was able to glean from both Ben and my parents the mental anguish they underwent at that time.

For me, even today, it is still very difficult to accurately describe my feelings while being 'put under' for the operation because of so much agitation, and of being terrified, realising that there was a strong chance I would not survive the surgery this time.

Going back to the operation itself, this second laparotomy identified an acute haemorrhagic infraction where approximately fifteen centimetres of the small bowel was removed due to necrosis (cellular death). In broad terms, bowel infraction is an irreversible injury to the intestine resulting from insufficient blood flow. This lack of blood flow usually results in necrosis, causing that particular part of the bowel to become gangrenous. When this occurs, it is a medical emergency because it can quickly result in a life-threatening situation.

In this case, the developing condition was associated with the first surgery for the ischemic bowel. In that surgery the twist in the bowel was correctly resolved by straightening, followed by a return of blood flow as observed by the surgeon. The bowel returned to its normal pink colour and hence the problem was considered resolved. Unfortunately, even with straightening, there were changes still occurring within the bowel itself which were not distinguishable or observable at the time. No one was aware of this potential problem until I became ill some few hours later. To resolve the issue of the haemorrhagic infraction, and as a life-saving procedure, the surgeon removed part of the small bowel to contain the spread of the gangrenous tissues and infection.

My next memory was regaining consciousness in the recovery room with my first reaction being highly emotional based on pure relief of having made it through the operation. This particular moment was without doubt an absolute mind-numbing experience knowing that somehow the damage to the bowel had been fixed and I had not died. Yes, there was a shorter bowel, but I still felt very thankful and blessed to be alive, thanks to the wonderful hands and skills of the surgeons.

In regaining some composure, my next response was the anxiety about the baby. My fear was that his life might have been compromised in the need to save me. My memory was looking directly at the attending nurse pleading for a positive answer, and when told that the baby is okay and that all was well in regard to both of us, there was a huge spill-over of emotions leading to a tearful reunion between myself and the little one in my body. It was, and still is, an incredible moment, and a point in time that will never be forgotten for the rest of my life.

Attached to tubes and other medical support devices, I was wheeled into the ward, and the first people I saw were my husband and parents. Evident from their faces were the clear expressions of utmost relief from all the anxiety and stress felt throughout the four hours I had spent in the operating theatre and recovery ward. It was clear that they had undergone enormous pressures, and some of this was now spilling over in their reactions as they saw me after facing the long agonising time I was in surgery.

Again, it is difficult to explain my own emotions on first seeing them, except to say that it felt so good to be able to see them again.

Alongside me in the ward was my obstetrician who had provided immense support to the family throughout this frightening ordeal, and seeing him was also very comforting. I was later informed that he spent some time before my return from the recovery ward reassuring my family that under the present circumstances the prognosis was good, and barring any unforeseen problems, such as the occurrence of an infection, myself and the baby would be fine. It was patently clear that those reassurances were a massive bonus for lagging spirits amidst personal anxieties, and I cannot thank him enough for the support given at such a crucial time.

In the process of regaining strength and composure, it was time to speak with my husband and parents about those moments of much trepidation. I felt deeply about what they had been put through, and as a sense of peace for myself there was a need to discuss, and where possible engage with and share their feelings as they struggled with all those fears and anxieties. This interaction was crucial because they were subjected to a high level of personal trauma, especially as they were totally unprepared for the events that had occurred over the preceding days.

Firstly, in speaking with Ben, it was important to look at the situation in the broader context, especially when realising that this current event was indeed a culmination of all the previous years of experiencing repeated corrective surgeries and poor outcomes. Through all the recurring events, he was always there to provide tremendous support in the belief that the next surgery would be the one to resolve the problem, and the chance of normality in our lives. Naturally with poor outcomes being the norm, and the repeated disappointments building one on top of the other, and the need to comfort me time and again, the failures had begun to take its toll. In this continuous cycle, Ben began to believe that the surgeries were becoming merely opportunities for trial and error, and in time he began to lose faith in the capacity of the medicos to find the solution.

More importantly, rather than enhancing the quality of life for both of us, Ben's view was that each attempt was in fact having the opposite effect. Each failure was acting as a drain on our willpower, providing no respite in physical relief and my general wellbeing. From his perspective this was a situation trending towards hopelessness.

Perhaps given all that had preceded, the high-water mark for him was the support to proceed with the total colectomy, believing that the removal of the large bowel, and the capacity to exist permanently with a stoma, was the best opportunity for us. As a testimony to the strength of his conviction, he also firmly believed that the removal of the bowel was the ultimate surgical intervention and a lifesaving option. Therefore, he was totally unprepared with any downsides that might follow, and went on to admit that it was clearly a false sense of security, given the events that had now occurred.

On the morning that I presented to hospital emergency, Ben, like my parents, viewed the situation as a glitch in what was a small setback. He was aware of the diagnosis concerning the blockage in the small bowel, and like all involved felt that with the conservative treatment recommended, the problem would be resolved, leaving me free to return home in a day or so.

On completion of the first surgery the members of the family were informed that the surgeon had untwisted the bowel and that all measures were taken to ensure that the organ was fully functioning again. To all, it was a relief, as the surgery was major. I was cut open right down the abdomen, but the procedure did not affect our unborn baby and the next stage was going to be a full recovery.

It therefore came as a surprise, and some nervousness, when Ben was informed the next morning that I was to be admitted for emergency surgery to address the problem of some further complications with the bowel. More worrisome was the urgency of the surgery, as the situation was now life-threatening. At this point he was mostly unaware of my general condition, and the levels of pain that I had endured. At that time, it was only my mother, who was a witness to the distress, who was present in the room for most of the period prior to the emergency surgery.

As the situation further deteriorated with two surgeries occurring within twenty-four hours, this turn of events sent shock waves through Ben, as he was suddenly confronted by a situation he had never experienced before. I asked about his thoughts and emotions, but he found it difficult to describe his feelings. It was all so tumultuous at the time. He talked about the many surgeries that I underwent, and about so much hope after each one, only to be left with one failure after another. He talked much about how he frequently observed the brutal nights as I underwent pain and discomfort, and of his dismay with the failures of so many of the procedures, making life increasingly stressful and uncertain. He lamented how this situation added further stress and uncertainty to his life.

Importantly, he indicated that while I was in surgery, his apprehension, anxieties and fear became extreme, in turn transitioning into horrible thoughts during the procedure, and later extending to the weeks of the recovery process. He compared these feelings as a near miss in a serious car accident where a fatality could have occurred. He realised that perhaps I survived the operation by just a whisker, and could easily have passed away on the operating table, leaving him alone. This was indeed a provoking scenario to deal with, and a very dark and troubling state of mind to endure.

During the surgery, he was very concerned about the life of our unborn. He deeply felt that if the baby was lost, going home to a nursery that would perhaps remain empty would be devastating. There was also the terrible consequence regarding the possibility of only the child surviving the ordeal. In this case, the thought of a child living without his mother was too difficult a situation to comprehend.

On the more positive side, Ben was truly honest when he said that his best reaction at the time was to lock all dark thoughts and outcomes away. He compared this to being in a position where on the other side of the door is storm and tempest, and therefore the best way was to shut the door and keep the raging tempest out. In this way, he is not always totally consumed by the horrible thoughts and potential devastating outcomes, even though he was aware that the situation was critical. So, on every count this event was one of the darkest days of his life.

Then it was time to talk with my parents about their reactions on the day of the surgery, and the weeks following the procedure. For both parents it was clear that the sequence of events had occurred at such a speed that they were also totally unprepared. As the situation worsened, each setback became very much like a sledgehammer to their confidence. Initially when the problem emerged, both were apparently quite at ease, believing in the normality of the situation as they reflected on previous incidents where such glitches were followed by a quick restoration to my normal health through the usual medical interventions. Therefore, taking everything in their stride, there was an understanding that there was little to be concerned about this time around. However, as each setback occurred to the point of being very alarming, there was a growing sense of trepidation, anxiety and fear akin to the sledgehammer effect I mentioned previously.

In speaking at length with my parents, there began to emerge the apprehensive feelings that they collectively and individually experienced. From the conversations, I was able to grasp the fullness and intensity of their anxieties in those two eventful days and critical hours.

Here are some of their thoughts which I would like to share with the reader.

On the day of the second surgery, my parents were informed that this was to be an emergency procedure, because the surgeons and obstetrician were very concerned about the rapidly deteriorating situation. This was relayed to them, and as the surgery was to be performed sometime in the morning, my mother, who was working as a nurse in the hospital at that time, was the first to arrive, waiting with me at the pre-op station. Having witnessed patients in distress over the years, it was evident that in this instance the problem was serious, and she fully understood the significance of the medical emergency and the presence of the crash team. Being familiar with the personal fears of patients undergoing medical emergencies, she comforted me as much as possible, and remained beside my bed until I was taken to theatre.

My father then arrived at the hospital and together with Mum sat in the café while the surgery was performed, waiting for word from the theatre on the outcome. In encapsulating their thoughts, I understand that there were a few scenarios running through their minds. From their perspective, the best result was if the bowel issue was only a minor carryover from the earlier surgery, and one that the surgeon would quickly rectify. In clearly wishing this would be the case, they both felt this would pose no danger to myself and the baby. However, in also knowing the operation was scoped as an emergency, they both felt that a more extreme aftermath could not be discounted.

In assessing the next move, their immediate concern was dealing with the possibility of terminating the pregnancy, if this was the only option to save my life. For them this was a position no grandparent would wish for, as a loss of a much-anticipated grandchild would be devastating no matter the circumstances. Both parents were reconciled to the fact that if this was the only option necessary to save my life, painful as it was, this would be accepted. In every sense there was little else other than to 'live' with the termination, and somehow work with the family through the pain and anguish tied to this decision.

The other outcome, and one that was truly frightening, was the possibility I would not survive the operation. This feeling was magnified by the fact that although at that time the full extent of the medical problem was unclear, there were some indicators that the situation was on the edge. This was centred around Mum's medical knowledge, enquiries that she'd made with other medical colleagues, and of course her understanding of the significance of the medical emergency.

Another factor that was worrisome was the short time between surgeries. Both parents were acutely aware that open abdominal surgery twice within twenty-four hours could adversely drain my resources and overall strength, so that my body might not be able to cope with the surgery. This was a real concern, as abdominal procedures of this nature can easily take its toll on a person. Putting all these factors together left them with a grim and apprehensive feeling. As well, having witnessed the many years of suffering through numerous surgeries and other medical interventions, the crisis at hand was brought to such a head that it challenged their usual sense of calm.

So, as the events of the day unfolded, my parents sat in the café facing each other, all the time absolutely on edge while waiting for word from theatre. Their main recollection of those moments was that neither could say much to each other, so as not to instil even greater fears of a possible worst outcome. Therefore, each was consumed with their personal anxieties throughout the duration of the surgery, and it was indeed some three hours of extreme stress for both, endured in personal quietness amid uneasiness and high tension.

Speaking with my father, he said that he wrestled with a multitude of incoming thoughts of how he would react if a terrible outcome was to transpire. He indicated that his extreme fear was that I would die in surgery, and he was trying to visualise how he would deal with this at a personal level. The thought of losing a child was never contemplated in his life, and he was now confronted with the possibility. His mind was thrashing, worried about how he would cope if something like this happened, and then extending to the next day, the next week, months and years. I do know that the one thing that was holding him up was his Christian faith, and to this end, he spent much time in prayer as I went through the ordeal.

As for Mum, when asking about her thoughts, she said that her mind was generally blank that day, and that she refused to contemplate anything. This is not to say that she was not concerned, having witnessed my reactions as I experienced so much pain. She talked freely about her anxieties as she saw me getting in and out of bed continuously, and pacing the floor of the room trying to battle the onslaughts of pain. Embedded in her mind was the constant plea from me for the pain to go away, lamenting the fact that she could offer no solutions as relief in those grim moments, except to rub my back and offer words of encouragement.

In the post-operative discussion I was able to understand her strength in working through the confronting difficulties. This was clearly displayed in the underlying trust in the medical team and in the surgeon, with the confidence being that he would come through, and that the procedure would be successful no matter the complications involved. Clearly, Mum had steeled her mind to think this way, and so dissociated herself from thoughts of any outcomes that were not considered useful. Within this frame of mind, she refused to think and talk of any other outcome other than me being okay. She felt it was better to say nothing at all while she sat with Dad in the café, as it was unproductive to discuss and dwell on matters that were beyond her control.

Very worrying to both my parents in the event of the worst outcome was how they would tell the rest of the family. To avoid any unnecessary anxiety, before the emergency surgery, my parents had decided not to tell my brother and sister, and the rest of the family, of the precarious nature of the situation. Even as events began to unfold in an unexpected way, both my siblings and other family members believed that this was normal routine surgery, and as before, I would emerge in one piece and ready to fight on. To turn this around and tell the family something quite different, particularly if it were my demise, this situation terrified my parents.

It was only late afternoon that my husband and parents were informed that the procedure had been completed, and I was in recovery, and I would be transferred to the ward in due course. For reasons that are not exactly clear, this transfer took longer than expected, which also caused some concern as my family anxiously waited, hoping there were no further complications.

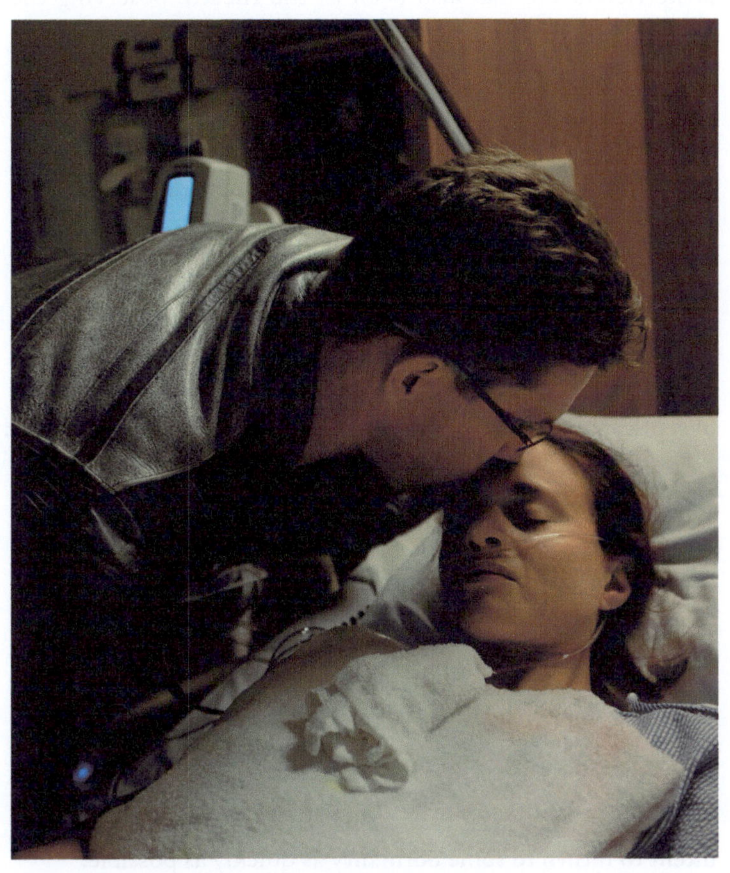

After surgery with my husband, best friend and soul mate (July 2017)

While waiting for my transfer, my parents and Ben spent time discussing issues relating to my early prognosis with the obstetrician. He had also been in the theatre observing the procedure with the interest of the baby in mind. Instinctively, the first question asked by the family was whether the baby had survived, and the positive answer led to immense relief. Alex, our first child and their first grandson, had also made it.

The other matter that Ben and my parents were told related to some of the more specific details about the surgery. They were warned to be mindful that the next few days were going to be critical because of other complications such as the onset of septicaemia. Clearly, I was not out of the woods yet, however, everyone in the ward that day was more than thankful for small mercies, especially as the outcome to this point was positive, and we were now in another phase. Thankfully, there was now a bit more optimism all around.

The physical healing process that followed was slow. This was primarily due to the length of the surgery compounded by the development of a wound infection along the incision. This was upsetting as it slowed the healing and recovery, and derailed my intent to return to some normality as quickly as possible.

In recalling this period while I was healing physically, I was in a mental state of some disturbance. I found it difficult to remain calm and relaxed for large parts of the day, and had great trouble sleeping.

This unsettling period while I slowly recovered centred on thoughts that were constantly in overdrive, mainly about the events that occurred during the day of the surgery. Deep inside me was a prevailing sense that the medical emergency was a close-run thing, and I was aware that as the surgeons scrubbed up for the procedure, both medical specialists were gravely concerned for my wellbeing, perhaps even for my survival. Certainly, the obstetrician was concerned for the baby, and the more these thoughts started to unravel, the level of personal agitation grew about the many bad outcomes that could have occurred.

Being very aware what had occurred in surgery, these events continued to dwell in my mind, as I was constantly replaying the dire consequences of the worst-case scenarios. I was now fighting the effects of post-operative depression, which I will discuss in the following chapter.

As I end this chapter, it is worth providing the reasons for my survival and recovery from two emergency abdominal surgeries in twenty-four hours. By the end of the second procedure, the physical impacts were quite significant because most of my strength and resources were drained, which could have put me at severe risk.

How did I make it?

I believe that the answer was largely due to the level of fitness that I had built-up prior to the surgeries. Fitness was, and still is, very much part of my life, even when battling through the many years of pain and discomfort. Maintaining a high level of fitness was always a core objective, an alternative pathway and effective hedge against the disease. As well, I used fitness programs as a distraction from the prevailing health issues, and to provide the strength to continue meeting the demands of life as best possible.

In developing a fitness regime, the focus was centred around a well-balanced tailored gym program known as the F45, which helped me maintain a high level of physical fitness through high intensity training. In these programs, the objective was to strive for and attain peak levels stipulated within the performance standards.

As testimony to this, I recall the occasion I visited an indoor rock-climbing facility in Fortitude Valley in Brisbane. The exercise included scaling a twenty-metre wall using ropes and other devices. Being fanatical in my competitiveness, there was immediately a challenge to my husband in a race to the top. Well, I beat him and this was no mean feat given that he was well into the martial arts of Brazilian jiu-jitsu at the time!

There is no doubt that in the years before the ileostomy and removal of the bowel, engaging regularly in a fitness program was much harder because of the increasing pain and discomfort due to incontinency. However, in the days, weeks and months following the ileostomy, my quality of life was much improved to the extent I was able to throw myself into gym programs, and achieve even higher levels of fitness. Therefore, immediately prior to the emergency surgeries, my body was bursting with strength, vitality and energy.

I am convinced that my high level of fitness must have assisted considerably in my successful recovery from the surgeries. Indeed, I received tacit confirmation of its importance during my discussions with the colorectal surgeon at the first consultation following the operation. To this day, his words will always remain in my memory, especially when referring to the concerns of the surgeon during the surgery. In confirming that the procedure was a close call, he commented that my overall fitness was very likely an important factor in overcoming the rigours of both procedures.

Perhaps it is a good opportunity here for some simple words of wisdom to those in similar positions, and who may be facing major surgery. While accepting that in some circumstances existing issues of mobility restrict the capacity to undertake fitness programs, my advice is that you should remain as fit as possible in the course of daily life. Fitness engenders a level of toughness and confidence in the individual, and therefore can act as a crucial resource in overcoming potential setbacks during major surgery and post-surgery.

Chapter 15

Experiencing PTSD

Happiness is not the absence of problems,
it's the ability to deal with them.
— Steve Maraboli

As mentioned previously, not long after returning home from hospital I started to become increasingly distressed, and my reactions were quite worrying to those around me, especially my immediate family. My body was recovering, but my behaviour was tinged with much sadness, depressive feelings and despair, even though I had thankfully survived a very difficult situation.

In trying to address my predicament by identifying why, it appeared that this was a delayed response to the recent events that had seriously threatened my life and that of the baby. Now the full impact of what had occurred was terrorising my mind. More particularly, some of the initial emotions of intense relief at having survived were gone, and were replaced by something a lot more sinister. In this short passage of time, as the relief from surviving the trauma receded, these new emotions and feelings established a condition I was most unprepared for.

As the focus began to switch to a different level, the one issue that seemed to rear up was that of recurring fear. Disturbingly, this all-consuming fear centred around the likelihood that should the twisted bowel condition recur, this time around I would die. Also, when trying to explain my state of mind, the most accurate description was that of a strong disbelief at being alive. This was kept active by repeated questioning as to why I had survived, when the logic centred in these confused thoughts suggested that I should have died.

In travelling along this dreadful and unproductive track, life become even more terrifying when I started to visualise the occurrence of another blockage in the small bowel. Thinking along this pathway was very much a vicious cycle, as dwelling on the possibilities of another blockage became a reality in my mind. In turn, this intensified my fears and had a compounding effect each time I thought about what happened. To add to the dilemma, and even more terrifying, was the realisation that the small bowel was the only organ left in my digestive track that would sustain my life. As a consequence, any twinge or painful bout would then trigger alarm bells that I was on the verge of a new episode, and another trip to the operating table.

Looking back, I realise it would have been so much more beneficial if I had the capacity at that time to recognise that these twinges were the processes of healing rather than fearing the worst. It is clear that a different approach would have calmed all my fears and anxieties by a factor of ten.

Associated with this regressive approach was my tendency to recall the periods of intense pain. I had vivid recollections of the moments before each of the surgeries, and the incremental build-up of pain as the medical problem continued to deteriorate that awful day. In particular, there was the constant replay of moments in the hospital ward, such as continuously hopping in and out of bed because of the unbearable pain.

Such was the intensity of the fear now taking hold that I was now convinced that in a recurring episode, I would not be willing to go through the experience again. In this state of distress, I pledged that the next time around, the inevitable outcome and fate that was in store for me would be accepted.

My thoughts next turned to the wellbeing of the baby, and being a nurse with some knowledge of the impact of strong medications on the foetus made the situation even worse. I was aware that leading up to the surgery and in the post-surgery period, strong pain medications were administered to curb the pain, and therefore my concern was the effect these may have had on the developing baby. My fears were mostly related to growth and development, and the quantity of these drugs the child had ingested, and their subsequent impact on the development of the brain. I reached the point where I began to review each drug that had been administered in a futile attempt to gauge their influence, all the time thinking this action could help ease the anxieties and resolve concerns.

Another terrifying worry was that the baby might have been deprived of oxygen during the long period on the operating table. In short, I was now totally consumed by the heavy burden of uncertainty and anxiety while desperately attempting to get back on my feet. Obviously, trying to solve problems in this manner is not constructive, and is unadvisable because of the unknowns that cannot be accounted for. Delving into the problems only resulted in continually living on edge because of the many unanswered questions.

As mentioned previously, I was also confronted by a setback with the surgical wound. For some unknown reason the wound did not heal as expected, which led to wound dehiscence. This is when the wound comes detached and the healing process is compromised. It looks terrible, but it is also a problematic health issue, one that requires immediate treatment to avoid becoming serious and even life threatening.

That further complication added to my current poor state of mind. Therefore, the bucket of problems was now not just full, but overflowing. Quick action was needed to rectify this downswing as it was causing a major setback to my recovery. I was able to seek immediate assistance from the local community health centre, which provided a nurse who visited my home each day to change the dressing, clean the wound and give advice on appropriate measures to advance the healing process. Fortunately, through sheer perseverance and good advice, the wound was stabilised, and I was able to tick this off as a problem overcome. For this, I am truly indebted to the attending nurses and their excellent skills, and a big heartfelt 'thank you' to all of them.

Recognising the need to address the issues associated with these emotive feelings of fear and dread, I took a pro-active approach, researching the impacts that traumatic events can have on the mental wellbeing of a person. As I delved deeper into this area, the essence of my feelings began to emerge, in that the emotional condition and reactions were not dissimilar to people affected by Post-Traumatic Stress Syndrome (PTSD). There was now a benchmark to work with, and perhaps an avenue to explore to counter the troubles of my mind.

PTSD is a complex area of psychology and it has taken me some time to understand the reasons why it affected me so badly. In assessing my situation, it became clear that my PTSD was being exacerbated due to my constant replay of events, and each time this occurred, it added to the mental anguish and invariably to the continuing downward spiral. This constant replaying also affected my sleep, and with less sleep each night, it was progressively regressive, further exacerbating the situation in a cyclic fashion.

I was at the end of my tether and urgently needed to find a way out of this mire. Frankly, I had no idea how. It was an understatement that help was desperately needed. Fortunately, this was just around the corner, and it came from the obstetrician at a regular prenatal check-up appointment.

I vividly recall attending the first consult post-surgery. The usual scans and other tests were undertaken to ensure that the pregnancy was going as expected. Happily, all the tests indicated that our baby was progressing well. This reassurance was a relief to hear, even though Ben and I were realistic in thinking that, ultimately, we would need to wait until the baby was born to be sure of a clean bill of health. Nevertheless, the positive news regarding the condition of the baby greatly helped in alleviating some of my concerns. At least for now.

After completing the usual checks, and setting my mind

somewhat at ease regarding the pregnancy, the obstetrician then said something that was visually obvious to him. His words will always remain in my memory for they were so poignant at the time and clearly reflected my actual feelings deep inside. Most importantly, somehow, and unknowingly, either in my appearance or manner, I had reached out to someone and the call had been answered. I will always remember his words that I looked 'so sad' and seemed 'almost broken and defeated'.

The obstetrician was really concerned about my mental wellbeing, especially in relation to pre- and post-natal depression. Knowing my medical history and the recent experience with life-saving surgery, and observing my general demeanour, he was singularly intent in negating any form of depression associated with the pregnancy and birth. Thus, he recommended that I receive professional help, and referred me to the Belmont Private Hospital in Carindale, not far from central Brisbane.

This hospital specialises in assisting persons suffering mental health issues and provides programs that suit individual needs. The core of these programs revolved around group therapy, organised within a setting where individuals were able to interact with trained therapist. More encouragingly, the centre had a high reputation for assisting people who had experienced trauma, using focused group therapy sessions as the tool to achieve meaningful results. I felt that this was an excellent way of combating my current anxiety and depression. The other bonus was that the hospital worked with patients who had pre-natal disorders, another reason for the referral.

The program required three sessions per week for six weeks

at the hospital. Without detailing the sessions, what stood out was the feeling of not being alone, as others were also facing difficult issues impacting their lives. In conversations within this shared environment, and aided by the special consultants acting as moderators, I was able to understand my condition better, and use the tools provided, confident in confronting the ongoing challenges.

Overall, the assistance and support the hospital provided was excellent; it definitely had a positive impact in alleviating most of my anxieties, and left me much more at ease.

A significant outcome of the therapy was its positive influence on my post-natal concerns. I now felt unburdened and better prepared for the birth of my child, due to be born in approximately two months.

While recovering, and using my new tools, it was now time to revisit my previous thoughts and behavioural responses, and better understand my reactions to the traumatic events surrounding the life-saving surgery. In the clear light of day, it was now possible for me to reflect on this period and better understand the strong feelings of anger, grief, intense sadness, and of course fear, which was the core issue of concern. With this in train, it was now time to reboot, gather up the positives, and slowly move forward to engage in the next phase of the journey.

That was the preparation for the birth my child. This was more involved than normal, due to the uncertainty of childbirth in regard to the stresses this would have on my body given my medical history. This concern was consistent with the early days when I enquired about ever having a child. I was then told that while there was no physiological reason for not having a baby, we were also entering unknown territory. To address these unresolved matters, including the impacts of the recent surgery and the stoma, specific health protocols, mostly initiated by the obstetrician, were put in place to manage the upcoming birth.

Foremost, and mostly as a safeguard against any undue strain on the digestive system, it was decided that the baby would be delivered by caesarean section. At the forefront of this decision was the recent major trauma relating to the twisted bowel. This had run up some red flags and suggested the avoidance of a normal childbirth, because it was unclear how the body would cope with these stresses. The plan was carefully synchronised and centred around specific milestones, always keeping in mind the need to look for the signals indicating pre-term labour.

In this synchronisation process, the initial aim was to ensure the viability of the pregnancy, and here it was decided that achieving twenty-eight weeks of gestation was the first critical milestone to be ticked off.

Beyond twenty-eight weeks, a strict regime was then followed with weekly monitoring using foetal medical scans to ensure that the child was growing normally, and on track. Consequently, as the weeks elapsed, and all signs of the pregnancy showed normality with each milestone ticked off with no hitches, I felt my confidence rising followed by happy expectation.

It was now time to wait for the big day and with it some critical decisions by the medical support team. The monitoring across the pregnancy and accurate timing became critical to ensure the caesarean section was performed at the most appropriate moment.

This became a fine balance between allowing the pregnancy to extend for as long as possible consistent with a normal gestation period, while at the same time avoiding the advance to labour contractions.

Living through these times, I was filled with a high level of expectation because of the advent of motherhood, but also very anxious because of the many unknown factors relating to the birth and condition of the baby. Naturally, I became very apprehensive on several occasions, although this was somewhat placated by the enormous trust and faith I had in the medical team.

With all the systems in place and the ticking-off each of the milestones, the obstetrician decided that as I was approaching thirty-seven weeks, the appropriate moment had arrived, and a Caesarean section was performed. On 11 December 2017, my son Alexander was born at The Wesley Hospital in Brisbane.

This was a wonderful moment for me in the light of the issues and challenges I had overcome to get to this point. In the time leading up to the birth, much had already been achieved, but notwithstanding these milestones, I still consider my greatest achievement was becoming a mum to my beautiful little boy Alexander. This was something I initially believed was not possible because of all the medical problems including the ileostomy.

My experience is the proof that living with a stoma does not mean you can't enjoy a happy and heathy pregnancy, and while my journey was a little more complicated, having a child was the ultimate prize and the reassurance of a normal life. So, for an ostomate this experience serves as a reminder that anything is possible in the context of their lives. Importantly, achieving such a milestone is so incredibly rewarding, but one that is difficult to articulate in simple words.

I wrote an article titled *My Ostomy Pregnancy* which was recently published in the journal *Ostomy Australia.* This described the journey of my pregnancy from conception through two lifesaving surgeries and ending with the Caesarean section. I make the point that in spite of all the problems, I would not change a thing, because the special gift of motherhood is so gratefully accepted.

At this time family was very important. I was fortunate to have at the birth of Alexander my aunt Amanda on holiday from Vancouver and my aunt Christine from Adelaide. It was wonderful to have them around to share the moment, and to listen and feel comforted for their continued support. The birth of Alexander was also an early Christmas present for me, Ben and the rest of the family. So, we set about organising our Christmas celebrations with the new addition. It was indeed a memory that will always be cherished.

After Alexander's birth, life continued normally until around the twelve-week mark when I experienced some disturbing but familiar pains. These set off some alarms. As usual, a visit to the surgeon was required, and it was discovered that some adhesions had appeared, requiring surgery. This was performed, and life continued normally with all the coping and learning about being a mother across the new year and through much of 2018. In this period my thoughts began to turn towards returning to work and resuming my nursing career. I planned to do that in the later part of the year, when my obstetrician declared me fully recovered.

And so, in thinking about resuming work, specific consideration had to be given in relation to the level of adjustment that I would have to make to fit back into the work environment. Much water had gone under the bridge. It was approximately eighteen months almost to the day when I had suffered the life-threating bowel obstruction, and I was feeling nervous about returning as a ward nurse. I was worried that by being out of the workforce for nearly eighteen months, I would have lost many of the skills I had learned in the first twelve months. It was indeed this lack of continuity that was particularly worrying.

I returned to The Prince Charles Hospital in late 2018, and while my fellow workers were very welcoming, my first days, and indeed the next few weeks, on the ward were somewhat difficult. This was mainly due to being tired, simply because my body needed to get used to the recurring eight hours of shift work, rather than the lack of skillsets, which was my initial primary concern.

In easing into my return to the ward, I must give special thanks for the support I received from the ward facilitators. They were exemplary in their patience and willingness to smooth the pathway. With their assistance and diligence, it became evident that my concerns and pessimism surrounding my absence were somewhat exaggerated. Not surprising, I was quickly into stride, regaining confidence knowing that my professional skills and standards were intact. Life at work was now back in full swing, and with much pleasure I resumed my nursing career.

It was also time to reminisce on all the years leading to this point, recalling in some detail the enduring struggles, and the intensity of the battles fought, and now thankfully won. In working through each step in the process leading to my recovery, I remain totally committed to the view that an ostomy is nothing more than an appendage to the body. It is certainly not an impediment to life. Indeed, it should be seen as nothing more than a short hiccup in one's life cycle, and not a limitation to achieving all of one's personal goals, as long as there is willingness, strength, and a preparedness to do so.

Being empowered by a new-found confidence, and having reached a pinnacle in my life after so many years of battle, I had the energy to explore and engage in many opportunities to assist others who have, or had, or are experiencing, similar difficulties. In this respect I also realise that being a nurse has afforded me the chance to enhance the lives of others within and outside the hospital network. I was determined to explore these pathways and commit myself to this cause.

Chapter 16

Celebrating a Sense of Victory

There are two ways to live your life. One is as though nothing is a miracle; the other is as though everything is a miracle.

— **Albert Einstein**

I am claiming victory over my twenty-year health battle – and why not? All those years ago, while still a teenager, I was left in a state of despair when denied many of the things in life that people generally regard as normal. Moving through adulthood, there was a prolongation of this distress while battling the obstacles and disappointments along the way, reaching a low point in the face of a life-threatening situation and then overcoming it. This claim of victory is for the opportunity that has been afforded me to live a normal and engaging life centred around the decision to be fitted with a stoma. Most of all I had a special victory in becoming a mother when seemingly this appeared to be well out of my reach. With motherhood has come the chance to live and share my life with my husband Ben and my wonderful son Alex. A small family, but truly a blessing.

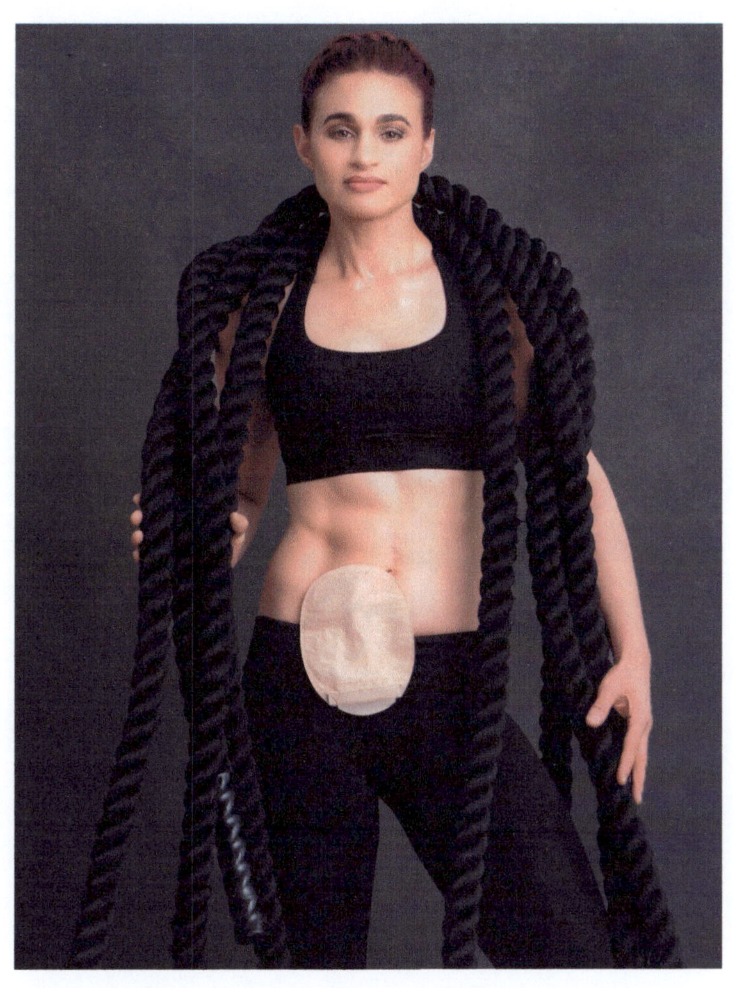

Celebrating World Ostomy Day (October 2022)

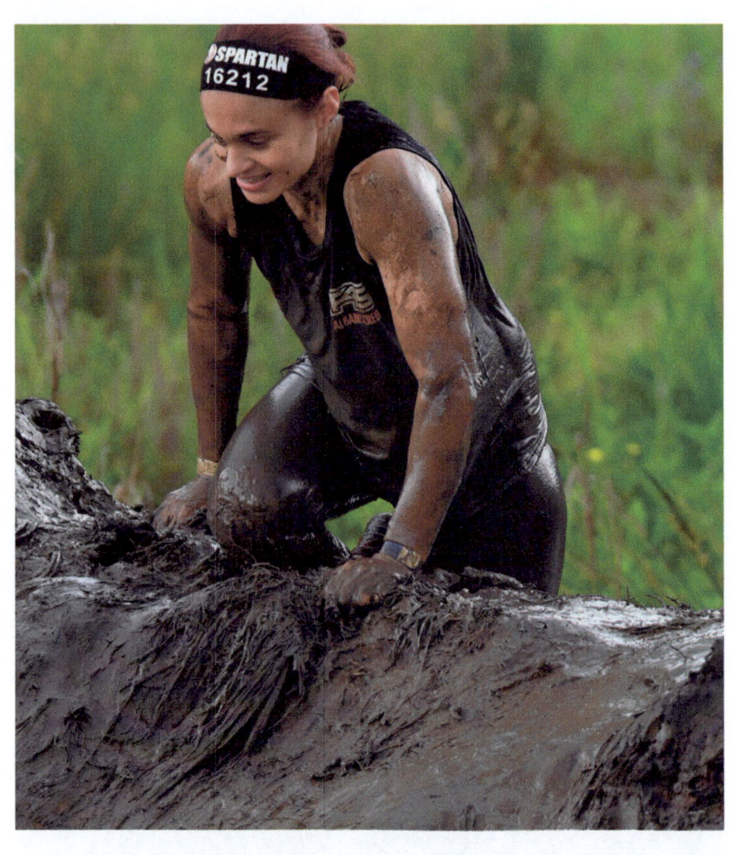

The rolling mud hills at the Spartan Race on the Gold Coast. (October 2022)

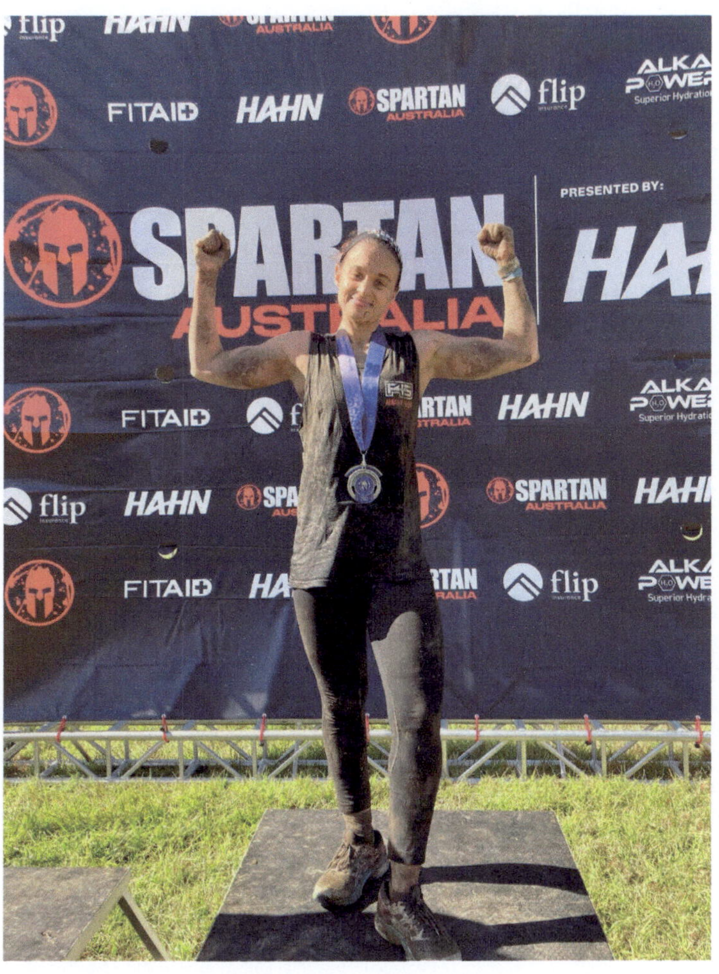

Spartan Race Finish Line after a gruelling 10 kms.
(May 2023)

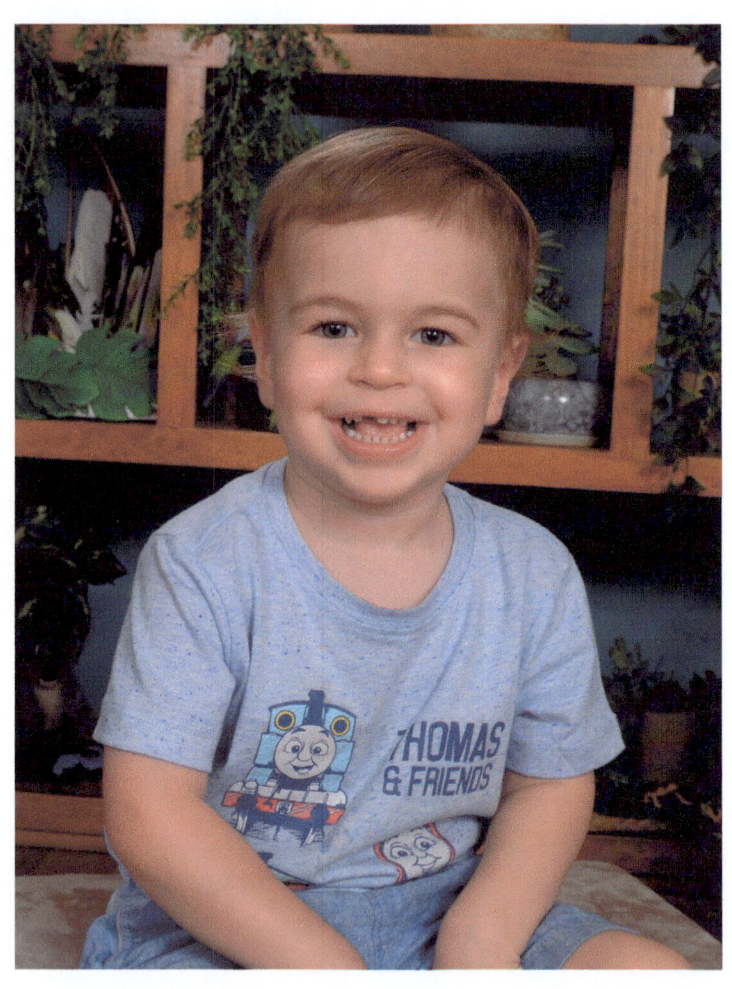

Kate and Ben's son Alexander at childcare (2021)

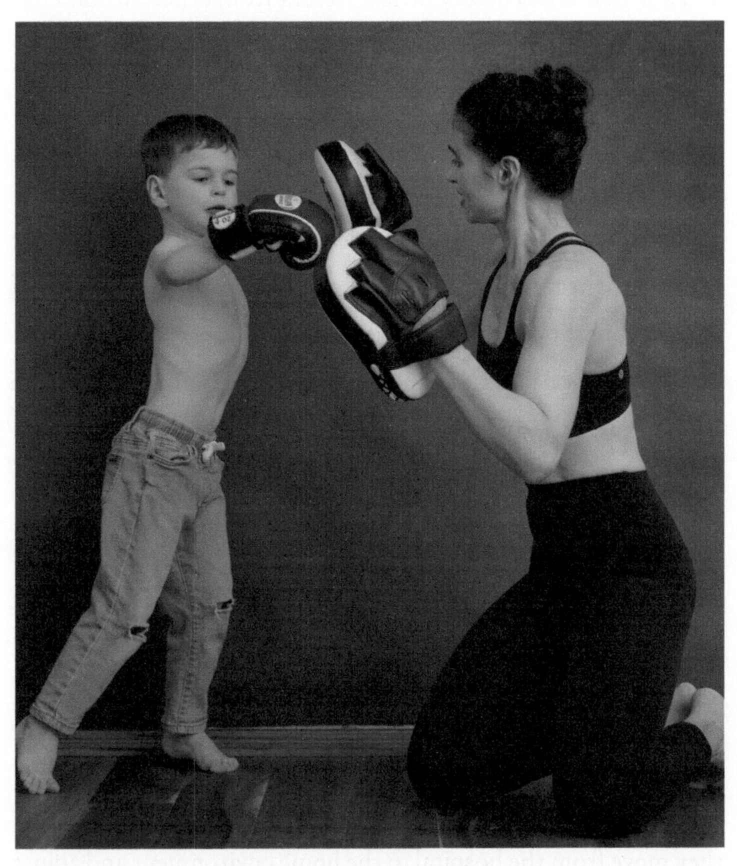

Kate and Son Alexander.(May 2023)

All the milestones mentioned above are without doubt tangible victories. I am now living a life never thought possible and one that is essentially little different from others around me. Importantly, I am living with what is only an appendage rather than an obstacle. Yes! I must admit that it sometimes gets in the way, but in reality it can also be seen as being no different to the everyday problems accompanying a person in normal life.

In Chapter 8 of this book, I described the difficult decision to leave the travel industry, which was then front and centre of my early life, and transition into a nursing career. This decision marked a pivotal point, and in every sense remains the right choice. It has brought the gift of tremendous job satisfaction, underpinned by the opportunity to contribute in an effective and constructive way towards the health of others and to those in my care.

In the early days after surgery, when life can be very challenging and highly emotional for a patient, I have been able to use my skills to explain the more finite aspects of living with a stoma, giving special attention to the importance of wound care management. As another bonus, there have been many opportunities to assist ostomate patients by providing advice as they move from the hospital to the home environment and adjust to daily life.

Full credit must also be given to the hospital in the positive way that stoma patients are being cared for. I feel so grateful for being part of this health care initiative as we send these people out to live a normal life in the community. The interactions with and ongoing exposure to patients have paid off in my increasing level of confidence, to the point where I can speak freely and with some authority on the subject, especially when addressing care from a nursing perspective. This in turn has had its own rewards, as within my peer group I am regarded as someone knowledgeable on the practical problems and challenges in the care of ostomates.

I therefore cherish the opportunities to speak at staff days and forums. In these events it has been full on in presenting matters relating to the care and management of people who have undergone an ileostomy or colostomy. I have used this avenue to gain a further foothold in creating more awareness about these patients. These talks also helped me to strengthen my base as an advocate.

I always use these presentations to focus on the clinical practices of wound care, hygiene and how to induce in the patient the importance of good personal management. Encouragingly, from the responses I have received from the forums, there is a growing inclination to bring about change, and therefore another step in the breakthrough journey to improve the care and management of ostomy patients. By using this platform to address a captive audience, there is always hope that by actively canvassing the issues, this will provide added value to the crucial work that my peers undertake in their daily patient care.

Importantly, and at the hands-on level, I noted that through these workshops, nurses and other medical staff were increasingly showing more interest in the emotional wellbeing of ostomates. Not being skilled in the areas of counselling, I am, however, very careful in my responses and interpretation of these matters, always trying to couch answers around my own experience, and the positives from the care that was given to me through all my times in hospital.

Within this medical setting when speaking as an advocate for ostomy patients, the information I present is mostly directed towards an appreciation that life for an ostomate is an ever-evolving situation. Therefore, my emphasis is that it is incumbent on health practitioners to keep learning and increase their knowledge as they become more involved with ostomy patients. It is noticeable that our efforts in the hospital have yielded positive results, and hopefully this will be the forerunner of a template to be used to inform others on building crucial relationships between the nurse and the ostomy patient. An effort worth pursuing.

A new area and another door that has opened since I started the workshop sessions is the relationship that has developed with the commercial sector – companies engaged in the manufacture and retailing of equipment for patients with ileostomies and colostomies. This includes corporations and smaller agencies that supply the tubes, stoma attachments, waste bags, cleaning equipment and other devices. Recognising this as another step forward and a worthwhile extension to the workshops, I embraced the opportunity as a further way to interact and engage with another group associated with assisting ostomates.

I have been invited to deliver presentations about my life and experiences as a stoma patient at corporate gatherings organised as workshops, small conferences and forums. Very encouragingly, these overtures have emerged through word-of-mouth recommendations from colleagues and medical organisations that have attended my presentations at staff in-service functions and other gatherings.

A most gratifying thought is that I must have made a good

impression on them about my ideas on the challenges, treatment and management of stoma patients. Setting aside the fact that some people may view me as being quite feisty in the arguments presented, it is still very comforting to know that I am someone worth listening to.

The audiences comprise teams from marketing and sales, including senior executives and support staff, and needless to say, these forums have a strong commercial element due to the underlying focus being the retailing of products. Notwithstanding the commercial element of these events, I am fully supportive of the activities of these agencies in their excellent work in providing assistance through the manufacture, distribution and sales of these much-needed high quality products. In the light of their crucial role, I feel no conflict of interest when complementing, and where possible assisting them, in their efforts to improve the lives of ostomates.

In the presentation format, I always use the forums to promote and reinforce the idea of resilience. In every sense, the message is centred on the importance for the ostomate to believe that irrespective of the prevailing circumstances, all is never lost and there is always a clearer road ahead.

In my interactions with the commercial sector, this message has also filtered through to the sales and marketing teams of the private agencies. It is so encouraging when the participants clearly recognise the importance of their efforts in contributing positively to the lives of people living with these medical conditions.

It has also been pleasing to note that at these presentations many attendees from the commercial sector have shown a keen interest in gaining an insight into the life of an ostomate, rather than just the clinical aspects of having an ostomy. While always acknowledging the importance of clinical matters, my life story, and in particular my enduring efforts to overcome difficulties against the odds, has been well received by the attendees. Indeed, it has been very reassuring to encounter such receptive audiences, interested in understanding the many issues that matter in the life of an ostomate.

I guess if my work results in a better appreciation and commitment from the marketing and sales teams towards improving the delivery and servicing of products, then these presentations have hit the mark. Indeed, when looking at the responses and feedback received, I am very satisfied with my efforts.

Another spin-off from these public engagements is that in some of the forums the attendees are also persons who are not directly involved in either the manufacture or sale of equipment, but are product users themselves. More particularly, these people have undergone ileostomies, colostomies or similar surgical interventions, and therefore are interested in listening to and contributing towards the cause. Having these people participating is an bonus as it provides the opportunity to interact and openly discuss the issues and solutions common to all who live with this condition.

My early engagements in speaking at private meetings and workshops were initially with a group called Liberty Medical, a subsidiary of Hollister, which is an independently owned company based in Chicago selling Densal and Hollister devices. The invitation to speak at one of their corporate meetings came about following my attendance at the Australian Association of Stomal Therapy Nurses (AASTN) conference held in Sydney in May 2019.

At this event I was approached by the company's territory manager who remembered me from one of the staff workshops at The Prince Charles Hospital. While attending a workshop, she was impressed by my presentation, and the message and emphasis in spreading the stoma message. She felt that I had something of special interest to offer that could be used to facilitate her company's work. Of particular interest was her belief that promoting a better appreciation of the life of an ostomate for those involved in marketing, sales and distribution could only be of benefit.

Etched in my memory, and an event that I wish to share, was the day late in July 2019 at the first of my presentations in a flashy resort in northern New South Wales. For that first speech, I unhesitatingly chose to talk about my trials and tribulations experienced over the previous seventeen years. More importantly, I emphasised the difficult life for a person suffering from bowel disease – the battle to stay normal over many years, and the eventual road leading to a stoma.

I spoke strongly about an ileostomy as an important respite that would lead to the emergence of a very improved lifestyle, and positives changes for the individual concerned, as well as for all those close to them.

This was the first of my ventures into the commercial domain, and it certainly had a very profound and humbling effect, which still resonates every time I make a presentation.

The unforgettable moment from that presentation was the reaction of the audience at the end of the speech. There was total silence, followed by a standing ovation, which continued unabated for quite some time. Looking around, it was evident there were many in the audience who were moved by my experiences. Witnessing such a reaction also had a very profound personal impact, causing me to become a little tearful.

In trying to understand how my words could have had such an effect on the audience that day, I would like to think that there must have been a thorough appreciation, understanding, and empathy in regard to my struggles and victory over adversity. More importantly, it appeared that the moment was not lost on many in the audience. The message was not just about me, but for all those suffering from various types of bowel diseases.

Stepping off the stage, I had this feeling of euphoria, knowing that I had indeed managed to deliver a poignant and strong message. There was also an intense sentiment that the impact of my words would continue to resonate in a challenging way after the retail sales personnel and support staff returned to their normal daily activities.

My presentation to the staff from Liberty Medical was a catalyst for writing this book. Following the session and during the refreshment break, there was a general discussion about my presentation, and how it would be useful to capture some of the information and supporting material that could be used as a resource. In considering this possibility, the concept of a book was then canvassed – an idea I had been toying with for some time. In further discussions, the representatives of

Liberty were also interested and broadly supportive. Although no formal commitment was given, there was enough momentum and encouragement for me to pursue this idea. There has been little communication with the company beyond these initial discussions because of the Covid pandemic, however, I remain grateful to Liberty Medical, to the territory manager, and some of their other staff for the initial support that has now led to the publication of *Overcoming Fears and Tears: My Ostomy Story*.

Following my initial forays into the commercial sector, the cliché that one thing leads to another certainly applies, as this was followed by another referral from Liberty Medical to speak at a community function as part of a local health care initiative.

This event occurred in December 2019 when a gathering was held in Tweed Heads in New South Wales. The session was organised by the Tweed Heads Support Group linked to the northern New South Wales Health Services. In preparing for the presentation, I met and liaised with Alex, who was a most gentle and resourceful person, thoroughly committed to assisting people living with stomas and similar devices. Alex and his wife were central to the work of the Tweed Heads Support Group in their quest to assist people like myself, and it was my understanding that Alex was also subject to a bowel disease and lived with a stoma.

With Alex's support and encouragement, preparations were made for the presentation, and in this instance his assistance was highly appreciated as this particular gathering was a little different from the earlier ones. Consequently, adjustments needed to be made to suit the audience.

This time, while those present included some industry representatives, the gathering was predominately made up of people who lived with a stoma. The reference to the stoma is used quite loosely here to reflect the fact that there were many people present who had been affected by other bowel diseases and were using aids such as colostomy bags. Hence, I needed to reach out to everyone in the room using the information as the catalyst to engender positive vibes for each individual.

Generally, the messaging was similar to earlier efforts in terms of my life story, but with the added focus on life as a young adult coping with the challenges of working full-time. I mentioned, as an example, the high intensity environment of Virgin Airlines. As well, details of my life outside of the airline environment were included, and the many health issues I encountered, culminating in emergency surgery. In this instance, I used the forum to encourage the audience in believing that nothing is impossible. I stressed that all obstacles can be overcome, and even though stomas can very confronting at the onset, there is an opportunity for a normal life.

Again, it was very pleasing to witness the reactions at the conclusion of the speech. I received questions that were positive in their manner, generally focused on seeking ideas and opportunities to improve individual lifestyles. An important part of the discussions was on new improvements in technology that would provide immense benefits for those with the medical condition.

I experienced a very touching moment after the event that is worth mentioning. While getting ready to depart, an elderly gentleman approached me with a gift that he had won in a raffle held during the lunch break. Having seen the delight on his face when he won the prize and stepped up to collect his winnings made it awkward to accept. I felt almost unkind depriving him of his good fortune. My first reaction was to decline the offer and thank him for his generosity. He responded that I was much more deserving of the prize than he was, explaining that my presentation had a profound impact on his thinking. He remarked on my fighting qualities and endurance over such a prolonged period of time, and said that listening to the presentation had rekindled the fire in him. Lost for further words and thanking him profusely, I accepted his gift. Unfortunately, I did not catch his name, but my understanding was that he was a cancer patient.

Such circumstances have convinced me that I am doing something good, and the direction I am taking is worthwhile. I think it is definitely valuable if the objective to assist others is achieved, even if it is by a small measure. This in itself has made me more determined to keep plugging away.

I cannot finish this discussion without remembering the gentleman, his kindness and thoughtfulness. To him I will say: *Thank you again for your kindness, and for making me feel I was contributing to the lives of many who were present that day.*

As a further note, while writing this book I understand that Alex who assisted and supported me in my presentation to the Tweed Heads Support Group has since passed away. Receiving this news really saddened me as I found him a model gentleman and a great ambassador dedicated to helping ostomates and others with similar medical conditions. I am sure that he will be sadly missed, not only by his family but by those he endeavoured to assist.

In continuing my work in the clinical sessions at the hospital, while at the same time making some inroads into public speaking involving commercial and other groups, another door in my quest to engage publicly with ostomates has since opened. Omnigon Australia asked me to write an article about my experiences living with an ostomy. Omnigon is an Australian company specialising in the supply of ostomy and wound care products to the Australian and New Zealand markets, and is similar to Liberty Medical in terms of its product lines. This time, the invitation came from the marketing executive of the company who, like others, had been present at some of the clinical presentations at the hospital, and believed that a contribution from me would be worthwhile to her company's magazine.

In pondering about the content of the article I decided to tailor my message around the issue and challenges of motherhood, given the birth of Alexander. This was indeed a perfect time to do so, and an opportunity to say that having a baby is viable for a woman with an ostomy.

Hence, I deliberately moved away from the experiences of my early life, and instead focused on the challenges of pregnancy. This article, *Being Pregnant with an Ostomy,* reinforced the message about the significance of motherhood and the blessing this brings to a woman, and that having a stoma should never be considered as an impediment.

My recommendation to ostomates when considering motherhood is to undertake research into all aspects of pregnancy for a person with a stoma, and to seek the advice of a gynaecologist before proceeding. This would involve the mandatory routine tests to ensure that the body is able to cope with the rigors of carrying a child, and childbirth itself, which I have termed 'the viability condition'. If this poses no problem there is no reason not to proceed.

In focusing on the details on what it is really like being pregnant with an ostomy, I have emphasised that a woman with an ostomy can indeed have a normal pregnancy, including enduring morning sickness, reduced energy levels, and discomfort. In my case, I mentioned that in the first trimester very few of the problems common to a normal pregnancy were experienced, and I was able to go about daily life much of the time.

Although I pointed out the normality of my first trimester, I did not refrain from mentioning the extreme difficulties I encountered. I did not shy away from the fact that due to an unlikely and rare complication of an intestinal obstruction, perhaps caused by an expanding uterus, I became gravely ill, with the possibility of maternal and foetal mortality. The two life-saving emergency surgeries in twenty-four hours were mentioned to confirm that there was always a level of risk in these situations.

The tone of the article, however, was positive, suggesting that while unknown complications could easily occur in pregnancy, childbirth was very achievable by women with stomas even under severe adversity such as a twisted bowel, rare as that was. I also briefly mentioned my struggles with Post-Traumatic Stress Disorder and some of the effects this had on my emotional wellbeing. While acknowledging that the psychological and emotional impacts of the surgeries and their aftermath played a significant part in my PTSD, I explained that this was eventually overcome by having good therapy with trained counsellors.

Overall, much of the article emphasised that persevering with the rigours of pregnancy provided the chance for an ostomate to bear a child, when at times such an idea seemed lost in a mire of uncertainty. The case here is my son Alexander who is an incredible and special gift to me and my family, and from my own perspective, to this world. Today he is a highly active, healthy and happy five-year-old and continues to meet all his milestones. This is despite my fears that there might have been some developmental issues as a result of the heavy doses of drugs and narcotics that were pumped into my body during and immediately after the emergency procedures. He is truly a blessing.

I have included two quotes from the article, hopefully as a source of encouragement to all those ostomates who are seeking motherhood.

Like any new mum, I still had to navigate through the sleepless nights and exhaustion, the rollercoaster of postpartum hormones and the difficulties of breastfeeding a baby that had trouble latching, but if you were to ask me today, I wouldn't change a thing!

* * *

Living with a stoma does not mean you can't enjoy a happy and healthy pregnancy and whilst my journey was a little more complicated for me, having a child is the ultimate proof and assurance of normality and a reminder that ANYTHING is possible.

It was not long after writing for Omnigon that I became involved with Ostomy Australia. This organisation's objective is to help people to actively live with a stoma. Thus, its main activities involve providing information about all aspects of stoma care. An important aspect of the work of this organisation is its promotion of stoma products such as care appliances and pharmaceutical products. As a user of stoma products, and as an advocate in supporting innovations and new technology in this field, I had developed an interest in the organisation over the years and welcomed any possible activities involving their work in the community.

Following some initial overtures from Ostomy Australia, I made contact with Kylie McGrory manager for Public Relations and Liaison for the Queensland Stoma Association. Kylie had seen my magazine article for Omnigon and felt that in the light of my experiences and personal trials, a similar contribution for Ostomy Australia would be very useful for its readers. So, in the middle of 2021, I agreed to write for its quarterly journal, penning an article titled *My Ostomy Pregnancy*. This was published in August 2021.[2] This effort was similar to my previous article for Omnigon Australia, focusing again on the challenges of pregnancy for ostomates. The article sits comfortably in the journal with a number of other articles submitted by my fellow ostomates on different issues about their lifestyles and experiences. Overall, I am quite pleased with my contribution as it provides a view on life's challenges from the angle of being pregnant while living with an ostomy. It is my hope that these articles will assist in

2 *Ostomy Australia*, Volume 30, No. 2, August 2021

generating more clarity for ostomates contemplating the joys of motherhood.

Writing for Ostomy Australia was very rewarding as this journal has a very wide distribution across Australia through the National Directory of Ostomy Associations. As well, beyond the local associations, there is also a National Directory of Ostomy Support Groups, which across Australia totals some thirty-eight member groups. With such an extensive coverage, it is clearly a most important organisation, with the capacity to communicate many ideas to support ostomates.

So, in this final chapter, with time to review and ponder about all that I have written, I keep thinking there is still so much more that can be said and accomplished. In relation to myself, my gratitude lies in being personally very blessed by having learned so much throughout the journey. It is truly very humbling to be able to present this book, as a contribution to the ongoing work of many who are actively working in this sphere, and of course those who have undergone, or are undergoing, similar experiences as myself.

Importantly, if my story, along with other efforts, provides even the smallest level of assistance in continuing the zeal to improve the life of ostomates, then much will have been gained.

In coming to the end of this book, one cannot go past the crucial lesson that is worth stating again, which is the need for an individual to commit towards looking for the best possible solution to her or his problem, even though some of the ultimate outcomes may not be totally palatable and even desirable. In pursuing this goal, the key lesson remains that when canvassing all options for a resolution, never allow setbacks to act as a deterrent. In this respect experimentation is the answer.

In my quest for living, learning and persisting, I owe much gratitude to many people who have assisted me in so many ways. It is through their efforts in helping to shape my thinking towards a positive mindset in the light of so many challenges that I am now living a life I am enjoying.

On reflecting on all that has happened, it is impossible to forget Karen and the role she played in comforting me when first I confronted the trauma of a life-changing experience. This might sound unthinkable to some, but when you see for the first time a swollen and red stoma, it really is a moment of despair. Yet there are so many knowledgeable practitioners who are available to help soothe and calm anxieties and fears.

When thinking of courage, how can Jessica Grossman be forgotten? The example that she set, not only in her country of Canada but for so many of us ostomates around the world, is inspirational. Recalling my discussion with Jessica mentioned earlier in this book, it definitely was her infectious nature and her drive to seek the best outcomes for ostomates that had a positive and profound impact on me. In fact, it was at this point that I began to take the small steps to face the medical challenges posed by my ostomy on life ahead.

I cannot end this book without stressing the importance of family and friends, and their support in shoring me up while going through the journey. I owe much to these people, and as a message to my fellow ostomates, believe unfailingly that there will always be bountiful support from family and friends as you go through your journey. And don't forget 'to get off your chair' as there is no substitute for fitness.

Most encouraging of all is the evolution in the management of ostomates, especially among nursing staff. One of the big changes is the increasing engagement between nurses and ostomy patients at a personal level. The net result is that nurses are now more attuned towards the broader wellbeing of their patients, an outcome so critical to the ostomate.

I am also witnessing a distinct improvement in the treatment of ostomy patients. While it is not possible to pin this change down to any specifics, I am inclined to believe that this is linked to an improvement in clinical knowledge, leading to better management and treatment. In simple terms, these improvements send a message to ostomates to look positively ahead, and with confidence in the medical sector.

I intend to keep pursuing key personal goals for myself. In the immediate term I will aim for a high level of competency in nursing. This will result in a significant benefit, not only in the overall improvement of skills to better assist others placed in my care, but a chance to focus on the special area of ostomy.

With the improvement in my skillsets will also come the opportunity to teach others in my profession about caring for patients who have different types of external appendages and other devices related to bowel diseases.

I feel empowered by working across information and education modules that provide contemporary data to support new ideas to assist in managing ileostomies and similar conditions. Adding to this area of research, information gathering and dissemination, my objective is to work at identifying and highlighting new technologies and innovations as opportunities to make life much easier for patients.

Finding ways to manage the emotional and psychological impacts of patients overcome with feelings of anxiety, fear, anger, uncertainty and even humiliation is a contribution that will also be very important. As someone with the lived experience, it is my belief that more opportunities can be explored within the clinical setting to improve the scope and level of involvement with these patients. So, my intention is to improve my skills in counselling by undertaking educational short courses on this subject. As well, I intend to supplement this knowledge by gaining more experience with patients and other professionals at the ward level.

Also included in this plan is the development of skills enabling me to work as a stoma therapy nurse, and hence my sights are set in obtaining a graduate certificate in stoma therapy. Overall, this is a two-pronged approach. On one hand the formal qualification will advance my recognition as being skilled in this area of patient care, and on the other it will provide the capacity for me to teach stoma therapy at a learning centre, which is something that is also close to my heart.

To commence meeting my goals, I aim to engage with as many people as possible to improve the needs and lives of those with an ostomy and similar medical issues. Over the longer period, coupled with the opportunities to work at different levels in hospital care, and gaining more competence and confidence, there is also the possibility of a career move, perhaps to the private sector.

And, most of all I am looking forward to a wonderful and fruitful life ahead, effectively ending many of the fears and tears of my life.

Epilogue

As I finish writing this book, we are effectively in the fourth year of the COVID-19 pandemic that has impacted Australia and the rest of the world. Sadly, with COVID-19 around I was unable to continue the work that was started inside and outside the hospital environment.

With the gradual return to normality in the hospital system, plans are now afoot by management to restart the in-house clinical and educational staff sessions. It is expected that soon it will be possible to continue the program of engaging with staff on ostomy issues, particularly in relation to the care of ostomates after surgery.

In the public arena, the pandemic had also made it impossible to continue with public engagements. At this time, with the welcome relief from the impositions of the pandemic, I am hoping in 2024 to pursue the initiatives mentioned in the last chapter. So, there is much to look forward to in terms of again engaging in clinical sessions at the hospital, and the recommencement of the activities involving the larger community.

Hopefully all of these opportunities will be in place very soon.

References

Western Gazette, Volume 104, Issue 98, 7 April, 2011 (www.westerngazette.ca)

Ostomy Australia, Volume 30, No. 2, August 2021

Omnigon Care Solutions. http://www.omnigon.com.au/customerstory/being-pregnant-with-an-ostomy